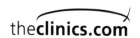

PHYSICAL MEDICINE AND REHABILITATION CLINICS OF NORTH AMERICA

Performing Arts Medicine

GUEST EDITOR
Seneca A. Storm, MD

CONSULTING EDITOR
George H. Kraft, MD, MS

November 2006 • Volume 17 • Number 4

SAUNDERS

An Imprint of Elsevier, Inc.
PHILADELPHIA   LONDON   TORONTO   MONTREAL   SYDNEY   TOKYO

W.B. SAUNDERS COMPANY
A Division of Elsevier Inc.

1600 John F. Kennedy Blvd. • Suite 1800 • Philadelphia, Pennsylvania 19103

http://www.theclinics.com

PHYSICAL MEDICINE AND REHABILITATION   Volume 17, Number 4
CLINICS OF NORTH AMERICA   ISSN 1047-9651
November 2006   ISBN 1-4160-3929-5
Editor: Debora Dellapena

The ideas and opinions expressed in *Physical Medicine and Rehabilitation Clinics of North America* do not necessarily reflect those of the Publisher. The Publisher does not assume any responsibility for any injury and/or damage to persons or property arising out of or related to any use of the material contained in this periodical. The reader is advised to check the appropriate medical literature and the product information currently provided by the manufacturer of each drug to be administered to verify the dosage, the method and duration of administration, or contraindications. It is the responsibility of the treating physician or other health care professional, relying on independent experience and knowledge of the patient, to determine drug dosages and the best treatment for the patient. Mention of any product in this issue should not be construed as endorsement by the contributors, editors, or the Publisher of the product or manufacturers' claims.

Physical Medicine and Rehabilitation Clinics of North America (ISSN 1047-9651) is published quarterly by Elsevier Inc., 360 Park Avenue South, New York, NY 10010-1710. Months of publication are February, May, August, and November. Business and Editorial Offices: 1600 John F. Kennedy Blvd., Suite 1800, Philadelphia, PA 19103-2899. Customer Service Office: 6277 Sea Harbor Drive, Orlando, FL 32887-4800. Periodicals postage paid at New York, NY and additional mailing offices. Subscription price per year is $179.00 (US individuals), $275.00 (US institutions), $90.00 (US students), $218.00 (Canadian individuals), $352.00 (Canadian institutions), $123.00 (Canadian students), $252.00 (foreign individuals), $352.00 (foreign institutions), and $123.00 (foreign students). Foreign air speed delivery is included in all *Clinics* subscription prices. All prices are subject to change without notice. POSTMASTER: Send address changes to *Physical Medicine and Rehabilitation Clinics of North America*, Elsevier Periodicals Customer Service, 6277 Sea Harbor Drive, Orlando, FL 32887-4800. **Customer Service: 1-800-654-2452 (US). From outside of the US, call 1-407-345-4000.**

Physical Medicine and Rehabilitation Clinics of North America is indexed in *Excerpta Medica, Index Medicus, Cinahl,* and *Cumulative Index to Nursing and Allied Health Literature.*

Printed in the United States of America.

CONSULTING EDITOR

GEORGE H. KRAFT, MD, MS, Alvord Professor of Multiple Sclerosis Research; Professor, Department of Rehabilitation Medicine; Adjunct Professor, Neurology; Director, Electrodiagnostic Medicine, Western Multiple Sclerosis Center; and Co-Director, Muscular Dystrophy Clinic, University of Washington, Seattle, Washington

GUEST EDITOR

SENECA A. STORM, MD, Assistant Professor, Department of Physical Medicine and Rehabilitation, Michigan State University College of Osteopathic Medicine, East Lansing, Michigan

CONTRIBUTORS

ALICE G. BRANDFONBRENER, MD, Medical Director, Medical Program for Performing Artists of the Rehabilitation Institute of Chicago; Assistant Professor, Department of Medicine; Assistant Professor, Department of Physical Medicine and Rehabilitation, Feinberg School of Medicine of Northwestern University, Chicago, Illinois

DAVID N. GRIMSHAW, DO, Associate Clinical Professor, Department of Osteopathic Manipulative Medicine, Michigan State University College of Osteopathic Medicine, East Lansing; Musicians' Wellness Team Physician, School of Music, Michigan State University, Co-Owner and Practicing Physician, Center for Integrative Medicine of Okemos, Okemos, Michigan

PAMELA A. HANSEN, MD, Department of Physical Medicine and Rehabilitation, University of Utah, Salt Lake City, Utah

NANCY J. KADEL, MD, Associate Professor, Department of Orthopaedics and Sports Medicine, University of Washington, Seattle, Washington

PETER R. LAPINE, PhD, CCC-SLP, Department of Communicative Sciences and Disorders, Michigan State University, East Lansing, Michigan

RICHARD J. LEDERMAN, MD, PhD, Professor of Medicine, Department of Neurology and Medical Center for Performing Artists, Cleveland Clinic Lerner College of Medicine of Case Western Reserve University, Cleveland, Ohio

THERESA J. LIE-NEMETH, MD, Director of Movement Disorders Rehabilitation, Spaulding Rehabilitation Hospital; Clinical Instructor, Harvard Medical School, Boston, Massachusetts

CLAY MILLER, MD, MFA, Clinical Professor, Performing Arts Medicine, Boston University Medical School, Peabody, Massachusetts

JUDITH A. PALAC, DMA, Associate Professor of Music Education; Coordinator, Musicians' Wellness Team, School of Music, Michigan State University, East Lansing, Michigan

LAWRENCE L. PROKOP, DO, FAAPMR, FAOCPMR, FAOASM, FAADEP, Associate Professor, Department of Physical Medicine and Rehabilitation, Michigan State University College of Osteopathic Medicine, East Lansing, Michigan

KRISTI REED, MD, Department of Physical Medicine and Rehabilitation, University of Utah, Salt Lake City, Utah

MARCY SCHLINGER, DO, Clinical Associate Professor, Department of Physical Medicine and Rehabilitation, Michigan State University College of Osteopathic Medicine, East Lansing; and Private Practice, Okemos, Michigan

GAIL A. SHAFER-CRANE, PhD, OTR, CHT, Assistant Professor Department of Radiology, Division of Structural Biology, Colleges of Osteopathic and Human Medicine, Michigan State University, East Lansing, Michigan

DAVID SHOUP, DO, Assistant Professor, Midwestern University of Health Sciences, Glendale, Arizona

SENECA A. STORM, MD, Assistant Professor, Department of Physical Medicine and Rehabilitation, Michigan State University College of Osteopathic Medicine, East Lansing, Michigan

CONTENTS

The health of performing artists may be affected not only by occupational risks but by concomitant illnesses and injuries also. It is essential that those responsible for their health care have an appreciation of all that is involved in performance careers, including the training, requisites for success, life style issues, and a basic understanding of the mechanics of each performing art form. This article briefly considers why the health care of performing artists necessitates a specialized approach and gives some suggestions for a modus operandi for success.

Neurogenic communication disorders are a routine component of clinical practice in physiatry. The organicity of motor speech impairments and of forms of dysphagia is a basic, recurring element of clinical practice in physical and rehabilitative medicine. The purpose of this article is to provide an overview of some forms of and causes for predictable dysphonias associated with professional voice use. Intended as a synopsis of hyperfunctional voice disorders associated with professional voice use, only certain laryngeal pathologies with functional etiology and their effects on phonation are acknowledged.

Focal Peripheral Neuropathies in Instrumental Musicians
Richard J. Lederman

Instrumental musicians commonly seek medical consultation for symptoms suggestive of entrapment neuropathies; the frequency in performing arts medicine clinics depends on the specialty orientation of the health care providers. In general, the focal neuropathies most common in the general population also are seen most frequently among musicians, although some specific differences can be identified. The diagnostic approach to the instrumentalist includes, of course, a careful history and examination; observation while playing should be part of the latter. Treatment in the musician is also similar to that used in other groups, but some differences may be dictated by the particularly high level of neuromuscular control required to play an instrument. Most focal neuropathies can be treated successfully, but further longitudinal studies will be required to determine the long-term success of current approaches.

Focal Dystonia in Musicians
Theresa J. Lie-Nemeth

Focal dystonia is an important neurological condition that can impact the careers of instrumental musicians significantly. Patients with focal dystonia complain of incoordination in their fingers or embouchure when playing their instrument. Abnormal movements such as flexion or extension of the fingers may develop eventually. The primary pathology appears to be in the somatosensory cortex of the brain. Several treatment methods are available, but results are not always satisfactory.

Common Musculoskeletal Problems in the Performing Artist
Pamela A. Hansen and Kristi Reed

In this article we examine some of the musculoskeletal injuries unique to musicians and dancers. The cornerstone of treatment in this specialized patient population is the understanding that the injuries these artists sustain occur in the context of a distinctive lifestyle. This lifestyle demands extreme physical and emotional stressors that are far outside the normal range of standard occupations and even most competitive sports. Understanding and treating all aspects of the performer requires a highly specialized interdisciplinary team approach that appreciates all of the conditions that govern these patients' lives.

FORTHCOMING ISSUES

RECENT ISSUES

VISIT OUR WEB SITE

The Clinics are now available online!
Access your subscription at www.theclinics.com

PHYSICAL MEDICINE
AND REHABILITATION
CLINICS OF
NORTH AMERICA

Phys Med Rehabil Clin N Am
17 (2006) xi–xii

Foreword

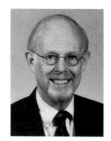

George H. Kraft, MD, MS
Consulting Editor

I knew a very wise man who believed that if a man were permitted to make all the ballads, he need not care who should make the laws of a nation.

Andrew Fletcher of Saltoun (1655–1716)

I am very pleased that Dr. Seneca Storm has agreed to act as Guest Editor for this issue of the *Physical Medicine and Rehabilitation Clinics of North America*, which focuses on performing arts medicine. Those of you who do not know Dr. Storm may not know that she is an accomplished musician, as well as a remarkable physician. She writes music, sings, plays guitar, and has done gigs and recordings. Consequently, she is well qualified to be Guest Editor for this issue.

The field of medical management of musicians' problems started in the early 1980s, and we are fortunate to have two of the pioneers as contributors to this issue: Drs. Alice Brandfonbrener and Richard Lederman. Although I do not know Dr. Brandfonbrener, I have worked with Dick Lederman over the years and am pleased that this outstanding physician and gentleman has contributed to this issue. In addition to these pioneers, Dr. Storm has recruited other outstanding physicians and clinicians as contributors.

Music medicine is not just musculoskeletal medicine applied to musicians. It also involves management of the changes in the central nervous system (CNS) resulting from years of musical practice and performance. The focal dystonias are incompletely understood CNS problems that do not involve the musculoskeletal system. These are also covered in this issue and are important for a comprehensive understanding of music medicine.

doi:10.1016/j.pmr.2006.08.005

I have long awaited this issue. Music is important to us as people and an increasingly important part of our practice. This issue contains the wisdom of the experts. We are indebted to Dr. Storm for gathering them all in one place.

Let the music begin!

George H. Kraft, MD, MS
Department of Rehabilitation Medicine
University of Washington School of Medicine
1959 NE Pacific Street, Box 356490
Seattle, WA 98195-6490, USA

E-mail address: ghkraft@u.washington.edu

ELSEVIER
SAUNDERS

Phys Med Rehabil Clin N Am
17 (2006) xiii–xv

PHYSICAL MEDICINE
AND REHABILITATION
CLINICS OF
NORTH AMERICA

Preface

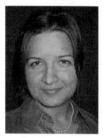

Seneca A. Storm, MD
Guest Editor

The field of performing arts medicine has experienced a great deal of growth and evolution in the last three decades. While Beradino Ramazzini summarized occupational diseases of musicians in his *Diseases of Tradesmen* in 1713, medical interest in musician's injuries remained limited until the late 19th century. The development of performing arts medicine mushroomed in the late 1970s and early 1980s. Alice Brandfonbrener, MD, organized the first "Medical Problems of Musicians" conference in conjunction with the Aspen, Colorado Music Festival in 1983. The conference is cochaired by Richard J. Lederman, MD [1]. This festival continues to be a forum for papers, demonstrations, and discussions as they relate to problems of musicians and dancers. Clinics, journals, and organizations, nationally and internationally, devoted to the care of performing artists has led to greater awareness among musicians, physicians, and educators. Resources exist within communities, and performing artists may access providers in their communities through internet sources like *www.artsmed.org* and *www.ifpam.org*. Historically, performing artists have tended to seek medical attention as a last resort. Thankfully, the medical environment that the performing artists face today is vastly better prepared to treat performance-induced injuries than it was a few decades ago. The climate Gary Graffman faced when he first recognized his performance-related injury, in which he felt "there was literally no place for me to go, and no doctor who would really listen to what I was saying," has changed forever [2].

The field of performing arts continues to face challenges, however. Myths about playing through the pain as well as fear of discovery for the

doi:10.1016/j.pmr.2006.08.004

professional performing artist who may face intense competition may still limit early treatment. Music education programs are working hard to create ways to convey the importance of medical conditions to a nonmedical audience. Dialogue among performing artists, musical educators and dance teachers, physicians, and health-related professionals must continue, particularly because many professional, semiprofessional, and amateur musicians have financial barriers to health care access. Appropriate education may help performing artists to prevent development or progression of performance-related injuries.

Performing artists may notice subtle effects of arthritis far before many other patients. The brilliance of their careers or the maintenance of their livelihoods depends on a reliance on a finely tuned neuromusculoskeletal system. As musicians age or develop other medical conditions that might interfere with their craft, they may need adaptive equipment and technologies. Adjustment to disability may be accommodating for an arthritic joint and modifying practice schedules, or it may be discovering a way to play the bass with a prosthetic right arm.

Over the last several years, we have seen increasing examples of functional magnetic resonance imaging as we seek to understand unique features of musicians' brains [3]. We are beginning to understand plasticity in the brain as it responds to music as well as finding differences and similarities about how musicians and nonmusicians process auditory information [4]. This search for the localization of musical skills dates back to the early 19th century, when phrenologists searched for the "organ of music [5]." This area of research may help us understand difficult problems, such as focal dystonia, perhaps while also advancing the knowledge of music and movement therapies as they relate to health and recovery from neurologic insults like stroke. Many musicians, both amateur and professional, developed a love of their instrument before onset of their disabilities. For those dedicated to the arts and music, physical challenges may cause change in career direction dramatically. However, in the pursuit of artistic expression, the only insurmountable obstacle is lack of imagination. Although performance-related injuries may forever alter the trajectory of a music or dance career, preservation of creative expression may have measurable health benefits [6].

In this issue of *Physical Medicine and Rehabilitation Clinics of North America*, we discuss specific challenges and general approach to the performing artist and dancers, common musculoskeletal and nerve entrapment syndromes, and movement therapies; osteopathic techniques and preventative strategies help us understand a general approach to the performing artist. Changes in musical education have resulted in increased emphasis on musical wellness with hopes of creating better communication between performing artists and their caregivers, providing care as an interdisciplinary team. Fortunately, performing artists have a great deal of information available to them. I am hopeful that we can continue to advance our understanding of difficult conditions like focal dystonia as well as limit injuries that may develop from hours of diligent practice aimed at skill acquisition.

I would like to thank the authors for generously offering their time and effort in this publication. Additionally, I am grateful to those who shared their libraries and expertise with me. Finally, I thank George Kraft for allowing me an opportunity to explore the world of performing arts medicine.

Seneca A. Storm, MD
Department of Physical Medicine and Rehabilitation
Michigan State University College of Osteopathic Medicine
B401 West Fee Hall, East Lansing, MI 48824

E-mail address: seneca.storm@ht.msu.edu

References

[1] Harman S. The evolution of performing arts medicine. In: Performing arts medicine. 2nd edition. San Diego: Singular; 1998. p. 7–18.

[2] Graffman G. Forward. In: Textbook of performing arts medicine. New York: Raven Press; 1991. p. vii–ix.

[3] Meister I, Krings T, Foltys H, et al. Playing piano in the mind- an fMRI study on music imagery and performance in pianists. Brain Res Cogn Brain Res 2004;19(3):219–28.

[4] Gaser C, Schlaug G. Brain structures differ between musicians and non-musicians. J Neurosci 2003;23(27):9240–5.

[5] Bentivoglio M. Musical skills and neural functions. The legacy of the brains of musicians. Ann N Y Acad Sci 2003;999:234–43.

[6] Barclay L. Music may be an alternative relaxation technique with cardiovascular benefit: Medscape Medical News. Available at: http://www.medscape.com/viewarticle/513790. Accessed September 30, 2005.

ELSEVIER
SAUNDERS

Phys Med Rehabil Clin N Am
17 (2006) 747–753

PHYSICAL MEDICINE
AND REHABILITATION
CLINICS OF
NORTH AMERICA

Special Issues in the Medical Assessment of Musicians

Alice G. Brandfonbrener, MD[a,b]

[a]Departments of Medicine and Physical Medicine & Rehabilitation, Feinberg School of
Medicine of Northwestern University, 345 East Superior Street, Chicago, IL 60611, USA
[b]Medical Program for Performing Artists of the Rehabilitation Institute of Chicago,
345 East Superior Street, Chicago, IL 60611, USA

Although each performing art has special associated risks, some are more immediately apparent than others. For instance, when actors have upper respiratory infections or sustain an onstage stage injury, the problem is unlikely to be life-threatening. If the show must go on, however, they may require immediate attention. A dancer with a severe ankle sprain will fare better if treated by an orthopedist familiar with dance, not because the diagnosis itself is challenging, but because optimal treatment and rehabilitation is done best by someone with an appreciation of the demands of the particular dancer's training and choreographic style and who is schooled in the requisites of executing the intricate maneuvers of classical ballet. In fact, being conversant in the applicable arts jargon is an essential first step toward successful medical interaction [1]. A violinist whose pain is limited to times when two fingers are simultaneously placed on two strings (a double stop) is evaluated ideally by a physician who speaks this language and is able to observe the painful maneuver with an educated eye. These case examples, while vastly different from each other, are fairly typical scenarios and provide ample justification for performing arts medicine as a specialty. It is critical to the good medical management of performing artists that it be conducted in the context of the art form.

Of these three performing artistic formats, theater, dance, and music, it is the musicians who historically have had the greatest difficulty finding doctors able to recognize their pathology. Dancers and actors tend to have medical problems more similar to those of athletes, which tend to be more readily recognizable even to the uninitiated. In contrast, musicians' injuries are often subtle and only evident in relation to performance, so that a physical

E-mail address: agbmppa@northwestern.edu

1047-9651/06/$ - see front matter © 2006 Elsevier Inc. All rights reserved.
doi:10.1016/j.pmr.2006.06.002

examination out of that context may be entirely normal. Lacking a full evaluation, musicians often have been assured there is nothing wrong, or, perhaps worse, in the absence of clear findings, have been given a diagnosis (eg, carpal tunnel) for which there is no hard evidence. Nevertheless, they are treated for the nerve entrapment they do not have [2].

Therefore, because musicians typically present the greatest diagnostic challenges, the discussion in this article largely revolves around them. There are common features in the medical approach to all performers, however, so that much of what is said about the care of musicians also applies to performing artists from other disciplines. Care must be timely, informed, skilled, empathic, and when at all possible, noninvasive. Other important common features are the long and intense years of training for proficiency, the need for constant maintenance of skills at a competitive level, and the fact that many patients are medically un- or underinsured. As a group, musicians are apprehensive of being diagnosed with career-limiting or -ending injuries, or treatments that will disable them. An injury often is misinterpreted as a reflection of their inferior talent, and they feel guilty about seeking help. For all these reasons, they are often reluctant to seek professional care, especially from practitioners of allopathic medicine. Performing arts medicine as a specialty is new, and in many places, both the artistic and medical communities are informed poorly as to the availability of such specialized care. This is changing, and artists are beginning to seek out performing artist practitioners, but many battles remain to be won, including persuading managed care providers that such referrals are in everyone's short and long-term best interest.

Because youth is not a protection against these arts-induced injuries, educational institutions and pediatricians need to be aware of the problems to provide the best care for arts students and ensure that their academic environments are consistent with maintaining good musical health [3]. Although there are some differences in health risks and factors to be taken into account between students, amateurs, and professionals, by and large these are differences in degree. So once again, for the sake of convenience, this article focuses on the special health needs of professional musicians, which in most instances will apply by extension to students and amateurs. An attempt will be made to provide some general guidelines for use in the assessment of musicians with medical problems not included in a routine medical history or physical examination of other populations. Other articles in this issue provide the details necessary to evaluate and treat musicians with specific symptoms associated with musculoskeletal pain syndromes, nerve entrapments, and movement disorders.

History

From the very first interaction between a musician patient and a medical care practitioner, there is a need to understand what the patient's musical life entails. Of special importance is a familiarity with some of the technical musical language, because often the presence of a symptom is confined to musical performance. Therefore, the patient can describe the problem best in musical terms. Although typically musicians' injuries are the result of the confluence of several risk factors, there is usually one particular event in their recent musical lives that represents the tipping point for the emergence of symptoms. Although the patient may spontaneously provide the needed information (eg, they were preparing for an audition and increased their practice time from their customary 4 hours per day to 8 hours a day), it may behoove the practitioner to ask the right questions. Thus an understanding of all the possible risk factors and precipitants for these musical injuries is central to being an effective musical physician, including some familiarity with the particular demands of each class and type of instrument. Many successful arts medicine practitioners have gravitated to this field, because they themselves have come from the ranks of serious amateur musicians, and their training gives them the insights to facilitate getting to the core of the problem.

It is important to inquire as to whether the patient has either had similar symptoms previously or has had other musically provoked medical problems. A positive past history of problems may be a predictor of ongoing problems and often provides some etiologic hints of technical playing issues including excessive muscular tension, poor postural habits, and overuse.

At the very least, questions should be asked concerning:

- Musical educational history (number of teachers, age at which study began, other instruments played)
- Job history, including current job satisfaction
- Equipment history (recent change of instrument, changes in instrument set-up)
- Practice habits (seated or standing, how long, how many breaks)
- Recent repertoire
- Rehearsing or performing schedules
- Habits, including exercise, caffeine, alcohol, or tobacco
- Medications (prescribed or over-the-counter)
- Trauma
- Psychological stress

Proper evaluation of what appears on the surface to be minor symptoms requires what is often a disproportionate expenditure of time. Moreover it is one that does not fit the current model for health care delivery. But, as Winspur notes, it is failure to take the needed time or to have the requisite facility for a thorough examination that has been responsible for most past medical mistakes in these musician patients [2].

Physical examination

Musicians presenting with pain or other symptoms that compromise their ability to play require:

- Complete musculoskeletal evaluation, including posture, strength, muscle mass, and range of motion
- Complete examination of the hands
- Neurological examination, especially of the upper body, spine, shoulders, and upper extremities

In the case of woodwind and brass instrumentalists who have complaints referable to their embouchures (the facial muscles, jaw, tongue, and teeth), however, those areas of the anatomy need the same kind of close scrutiny given to the body as a whole in players of nonblown instruments. Limiting the examination to the upper extremity with pain often will result in an inaccurate diagnosis and consequently the institution of inappropriate therapy. Failure to undress a patient and make complete observations of, for instance, winged scapulas, can be responsible for missing the most important findings and therefore a lack of understanding of what is the basis for a musician's poor posture with an instrument and consequent upper extremity symptoms [4]. Whereas there may be distal tendonitis in the forearm of a musician, the underlying cause of this problem may be inefficient body mechanics used in playing the instrument because of poor proximal postural habits or because of a lack of endurance in the larger muscle groups of the shoulder and upper back. If one does not look for the possibility of these kinds of findings by making a full examination, one may be none the wiser for what has been missed until weeks later when therapy for the more distal arm problem fails.

There are other physical characteristics of some musicians that may increase their risk for injuries. These range from physical dimensions including short or tall stature, relative arm segment length, and hand size features that may produce challenging disproportions between the musician and his or her instrument, or the demands of certain repertoire. Likewise joint characteristics, especially of the fingers, with either abnormally increased or decreased range of motion, may contribute to difficulties negotiating the keys or strings of a particular instrument. Instruments are generally designed for a limited range of body variability, which is for an arbitrarily average or normal hand configuration. Joints with genetically excessive range of motion and unstable finger joints (joint laxity or double jointedness) may cause the musician to compensate consciously or unconsciously with increased muscle tension in an attempt to stabilize the finger on a key or string, leading to muscular stress and tendonitis.

The unique aspect of the physical examination as performed by performing arts medicine practitioners is that of the patient with his or her musical instrument. There are some important caveats in performing and interpreting this examination. No matter how familiar the examiner may be with the instrument played by his/her patients, medical licensure does not include expertise in musical pedagogy. A study by Ackermann and Adams demonstrates the lack of interobserver reliability in examining the posture and musculoskeletal system of musicians. When the physical therapists surveyed, however, were also at home with the physical demands imposed by playing the violin, the consistency of their evaluations was improved significantly [5]. A medical practitioner can learn from careful and repeated observation of musicians, their patients and nonpatients, about the range of possibilities in requisite posture and the mechanics of musical performance. Nonmusicians can observe awkward positions, ergonomically questionable postures or maneuvers, inappropriate muscle tension, and physical misuse and abuse. Therefore, while musical criticism is definitely inappropriate, careful and sensitive questioning about posture and technique by a medically trained person is legitimate, and the insights gained by both musician and therapist can provide the basis for understanding the origins of a physical symptom and therefore for determining an effective strategy for its resolution.

The more opportunities one has to observe musicians, the more one learns and the more insightful are one's observations. These learning times need not be confined to the examining room. Every concert attended is a potential classroom for the medical practitioner. There are also opportunities provided by conservatories and summer music festivals, where the public may attend master classes. These sessions provide an opportunity to witness teaching by experienced and successful performers and musical pedagogues of their often talented music students.

Treatment of musicians

Specific treatment regimens for certain of the more commonly encountered musicians' problems are discussed elsewhere in detail. There are some general principles, however, that may be helpful to highlight in this article.

All patients are sensitive to issues of confidentiality, but this is especially true, in the author's experience, when dealing with musicians. One reason is that they may feel, often with justification, that if potential employers or even their peers become aware of an impairment, they will be passed up for work. In an area where there tend to be many more talented musicians than there are work opportunities, it is the physician's obligation to ensure support of them in any way possible, including protecting their right to privacy regarding medical information. Even a chance meeting of a colleague in the waiting room may be discomfiting, and physicians need to be on guard that information is not disclosed carelessly. This includes dealing with phone calls from managers or others who have a vested interest in the health of these musicians, no matter how altruistic the inquiry may appear to be on the surface. It is the patient's responsibility to share or not share any information with whosoever he or she may choose, and they need to be reassured that physicians will not disclose any information without specific their permission. The author extends this to a policy of not making decisions for musician patients as to whether to cancel a performance, or play a particular service, or of the length of their absences from work. The attempt is made to give patients the information they need to make appropriate and informed decisions. With their permission, the author will talk to personnel managers or teachers, and often will try to help an orchestral musician ease back into work with some kind of a graduated schedule for reactivation.

With the possible exception of acute coincidental trauma, it is important to remember that very few of the medical problems of musicians represent true medical emergencies. Therefore, even in the face of an impatient patient (and they frequently are), it is important to recognize how frightened these people are, and that in the long run, they generally will fare better when invasive procedures are at least preceded by a trial of medically conservative, noninvasive treatment. Rightly or wrongly, most musicians regard the scalpel as a threat to their career. Although this fear is rarely realistic, it is their perception, and in most instances, the problems they have do not make them candidates for surgery. Musicians are extremely sensitive to minor decrements of function and comfort, and their high level of performance depends on their ease, physically and psychologically. If surgery is contemplated in a musician, it should be done only for well-established diagnoses and never to explore for some poorly documented source of symptoms [6].

One of the challenges and opportunities involved in the practice of performing arts medicine is that the evaluation and treatment of these patients often involves expertise that spans several medical specialties and necessitates input from other artists or teachers of the arts. One never should hesitate to work as part of a team in the care of these patients, not only to provide improved care, but also for the learning opportunities provided to all the participants in the dialog. Assembling a group of dedicated medical specialists in such fields as physical medicine, neurology, internal medicine, otolaryngology, and psychiatry is usually an essential feature of providing optimal care at a performing arts clinic.

Medical practitioners who understand the complexity of these patients and their problems will find that their care is time-intensive compared with many other groups of patients, and 10 to 15 minutes of office time will not come close to sufficing. Performing artists are challenging, fascinating, and occasionally antagonistic. The process of their care can be frustrating to patients and physicians alike. Musicians likewise, however, often are surprised and grateful when their complaints are taken seriously, and they are treated empathically and with dignity, assurance, and reassurance. If their problem is resolved, their pain is eased and they are returned as expeditiously as possible to what they love and do best, they will be eternally grateful, and practitioners will have the dual gratification of medical success and the potential for increased musical satisfaction.

References

[1] Brandfonbrener A. From the editor. Doctor/patient communication for dummies. Med Probl Perform Art 2003;18(2):1–2.
[2] Winspur I. Advances in objective assessment of hand function and outcome assessment of the musician's hand. Hand Clin 2003;19:483–93.
[3] Burkholder K, Brandfonbrener A. Performance-related injuries among student musicians at a specialty clinic. Med Probl Perform Art 2004;19(3):116–22.
[4] Wynn-Parry C. The musician's arm and hand pain. In: Winspur I, Wynn-Parry C, editors. The Musician's hand: a clinical guide. London: Martin Dunitz; 1998. p. 5–12.
[5] Ackermann B, Adams R. Interobserver reliability of general practice physiotherapists in rating aspect of the movement patterns of skilled violinists. Med Prob Perform Art 2004;19(1): 3–11.
[6] Amadio P. Surgical assessment of musicians. Hand Clin 2003;19:241–6.

ELSEVIER
SAUNDERS

Phys Med Rehabil Clin N Am
17 (2006) 755–760

PHYSICAL MEDICINE
AND REHABILITATION
CLINICS OF
NORTH AMERICA

Care of the Vocalist: An Uncommon Perspective in Rehabilitative Medicine

Peter R. LaPine, PhD, CCC-SLP

*Department of Communicative Sciences and Disorders, Michigan State University,
215 Oyer Clinic, East Lansing, MI 48824, USA*

By some definition, nearly everyone reading this article is a professional voice user. By virtue of the disciplines practiced, nearly everyone uses human voice as a primary method of transmitting information in their daily professional routine. Sometimes this oral transmittal happens under duress; even at times under extreme stress. In other environs, it might be transmitted in lighthearted, friendly banter. There are, of course, individuals who use their voices as an instrument of their occupation. Those individuals whose voices are part of their livelihood are generally professional vocalists, including singers, actors, politicians, and broadcasters and members of other similar occupations [1,2]

Professional voice use relies essentially upon the balanced relationship between at least three of the speech processes: respiration, phonation, and resonance. An imbalance among these processes when brought about by physical demands or personal habits can lead to various well-known, clinically recognized voice disorders.

This article identifies some of the changes in phonation that are associated with performing arts, with particular emphasis on the relevance for physical medicine and rehabilitation. Issues surrounding performance anxiety are not included within the realm of behavioral voice disorders per se.

Generally, the subjective, perceptual estimates of human voice can be divided into three characteristics: vocal pitch, vocal loudness, and vocal quality. The listener's perception of pitch is associated with recognition of the tone produced—high pitch, neutral, or low pitch. Loudness is a subjective category relative to the listener's perception of the speech signal. Quality is an obtuse perception that is subject to considerable debate and difficult to operationally define. This subjective element is recognized generally as any variation in vocal tone produced; the descriptors for these variations

E-mail address: lapine@msu.edu

1047-9651/06/$ - see front matter © 2006 Elsevier Inc. All rights reserved.
doi:10.1016/j.pmr.2006.06.004

can range along a continuum from hoarse to harsh, or even a breathy quality. Thus, the parameter of adequate vocal quality implies the consistency and ease of vocal fold vibration that produces what is acceptable to the listener as clear vocal tone.

Objective measures to evaluate pitch loudness and quality are available [3,4]; however, the reliability and validity of such measures is always an important consideration. Because pitch is the perceptual estimate, a measurement of Fundamental Frequency (F0) in the time domain can be determined for the vocal fold vibration during a given segment of phonation. Loudness is a psychological correlate of vocal intensity; thus, intensity as measured in the amplitude domain, such as a referent in the decibel scale. Waveform, the psychological correlate of vocal quality, can be measured relative to spectral display as variations of frequency perturbation and amplitude perturbation. Quantification of vocal parameters is not the focus of this writing; however, additional information can be found in Verdolini and Titze [5].

Phonatory characteristics of professional voice users involve applied aspects of acting, aesthetics, role play, personality factors, performance demands, psychological variables, pre-and postperformance routines, and reasonable vocal hygiene. These characteristics place vocalists under circumstances that may induce prolonged periods of use-related vocal abuse or misuse, conceivably in problematic settings with less than ideal acoustics, leading to alterations in vocal technique. As a result, these circumstances may produce phonatory conditions that cause the vocal folds to change, then subsequently with continued use, they can deteriorate structurally. The physical deterioration may be initiated by vocal fatigue, followed by laryngeal discomfort. Continued misuse will lead to vocal fold edema; the effect of this sequence may produce perceptual changes in pitch, loudness, and vocal quality, which in turn instigate compensatory techniques to produce clearer voicing. These compensatory techniques preface the functional or hyperfunctional voice changes, which manifest the consummate effect: an audible change in voicing, dysphonia.

Aphonia and dysphonia are forms of voice disorders. A voice disorder is any deviation in pitch, loudness, quality, or other basic vocal attribute that consistently interferes with communication, draws unfavorable attention, adversely affects the speaker or the listener, or is inappropriate to age, gender, and perhaps the culture or class of the individual. It may be organic or functional in nature and may be the result of laryngeal function or resonance disorders [6]. Inherent in the performance arts is the probable vulnerability of functional voice disorders. Organic voice disorders, however, may occur. The most prevalent functional voice disorders are those that are use-related such as the hyperfunctional voice disorders resulting from benign lesions of additive mass: vocal nodules and vocal polyps.

Vocal nodules and polyps are lesions associated with voice abuse or misuse. In the case of professional voice users, conditions of abuse or misuse can coexist. Abuse, typically speech-related, may stem from a prolonged performances or extensive rehearsals; misuse, or nonspeech related, may occur as a result of negative behaviors such as reactive airway, allergy, postnasal drip and throat clearing or performance-linked activities like character impersonations. These growths develop anatomically on the junction of the anterior and middle third of the true vocal fold and are visualized with endoscopic technique. Perceptual characteristics associated with voices affected by vocal nodules or vocal polyps are similar. The qualitative changes in voicing are: hoarseness, low pitch, breathiness, and, not surprisingly, globus sensation.

Vocal nodules are callous-like, localized collections of keratin tissue associated with recurring vocal fold trauma. Vocal polyps tend to be focal, soft, pliable, gelatinous growths equally traumatic to the vocal fold yet known to occur after a singular trauma to the glottal margins. Vocal nodules tend to occur bilaterally on the true vocal fold; vocal polyps are often unilateral. Either lesion will cause added vocal fold mass and will create a glottal chink anterior to and posterior from the lesion. Hence, added mass of the vocal fold may produce a lower vibratory rate, giving the perceptual characteristic of lower pitch. The glottal chink allows for air escape because of the inadequate vocal fold approximation causing the perception of breathy voice quality. Acoustically, the lower pitch can be measured as lower fundamental frequency; the breathy quality can be evident as a component of frequency perturbation or in the signal-to-noise ratio.

These two common forms of vocal fold pathology tend to develop sequentially. Initially, aggressive vocal fold approximation leads to the onset of edema. This edema creates the somatosensory impetus for the speaker to increase respiratory effort in an attempt to regulate unwanted changes in vocal pitch and quality [7]. This compensation perpetuates the pattern of hyperkinetic vocal fold vibration, leading to the physical breakdown of the free margin of the vocal fold microscopically.

Effective management of such lesions involves elimination of the causal behavior or the source of the phonotrauma [8,9]. Management techniques include differential diagnoses based upon behavioral analysis, objective assessment of vocal characteristics, perceptual assessment, and, if necessary, symptomatic voice therapy. In some cases, microlaryngoscopy with excision followed by a brief course of voice therapy may be warranted.

Other considerations affecting professional voice users that result from vocal abuse or misuse include the concussive effects of coughing and swelling associated with acute laryngitis, allergies, and sinus problems, including postnasal drip and medications, for their propensity to cause contact granuloma. Medications that dry the laryngeal mucosa, such as decongestants and antihistamines, should be noted.

Prevalent among all age groups and yet evident in the lifestyles and personalities associated with professional voice use is the concern for gastroesophageal reflux disease (GERD) [7]. Associated with the weakening of the upper or lower esophageal sphincter, GERD as related to voice use contributes to erythema within the laryngeal vestibule, primarily within the interarytenoid space. There is, however, a characteristic effect on the phonation secondarily. Vocal quality is compromised with the key perceptual feature of hoarse voice quality, or the diagnosis of dysphonia secondary to GERD. Management strategies for GERD include changes in diet and lifestyle. Further, symptomatic management can be accomplished with medications, including H2 blockers, and proton pump inhibitors. In cases when changes in diet, lifestyle, or use of proper medications are not successful in controlling the symptoms of GERD, surgical procedures such as fundoplication may be required.

Of particular importance to professional voice users relative to GERD are the contraindications of reflux medications, as such medications can exacerbate the colonization of *Candida albicans* [10,11]. *Candida* can disrupt the vibratory characteristics of the superficial layer of the vocal folds. This colonization may alter the somatosensory perception of the voice user, leading to compensatory behaviors that change vocal production. GERD is a critical issue for professional voice users; efforts to eliminate GERD should be stressed routinely.

An important aspect related to working clinically with professional voice users is to make the distinction between vocalists who sing for personal enjoyment as opposed to those individuals who sing and perform as part of their economic livelihood. Clinical recommendations regarding voice therapy, and stressing vocal technique may be dependent upon this distinction [12]. Individuals who use their voices for their economic livelihood face immediate ramifications if they are unable to perform. Individuals who sing for enjoyment may not be interested in additional income, but may use the performances as measures of social or personal value. Therefore, the need for a careful case history and personal interview cannot be understated. Psychophysical scaling instruments may be helpful to determine the psychodynamic impact of voice use [13,14]. For example, Jacobson and colleagues developed an index to quantify the psychological effects of voice difficulties [15]. The Voice Index (VHI) allows for measurement of emotional, functional, and physical estimates of voice use. The VHI is available for singers, and there is a Spanish version [16].

Ideally, professional voice users are managed most efficiently in the context of team care. This team can include various professionals, such as an otolaryngologist, speech language pathologist, a psychologist, and a trained singer—preferably a member of the National Association of Teachers of Singing (NATS). Such teams frequently are located in metropolitan areas or associated with clinical practices devoted to otolaryngology and voice-related issues. The American Speech Language and Hearing Association provides a resource for locating specialists in the area of voice disorders. Special Interest Group 3, Voice and Voice Disorders, is sponsored by the University of Iowa Department of Head/Neck Surgery. Its purpose is "is to promote discussion among health care professionals, scientists, and professional voice users regarding clinical and scientific issues relating to the normal and disordered human voice" (Available at: http://www.asha.org/about/membership-certification/divs/d3list.htm).

For obvious reasons, many professional voice users will need to seek out a medical opinion from an otolaryngologist initially; the physician may refer resources more familiar with management of phonatory issues associated with professional voice. In addition to the medical examination, the evaluation could include videostroboscopy to examine and document vocal fold motility and function, computer-assisted acoustic evaluation, and a perceptual analysis. Speech language pathologists trained in voice disorders should have academic and clinical backgrounds relevant to perform videostroboscopic examination with proper endoscopic technique [17], computer-assisted acoustic analysis, and the perceptual evaluation [3,18,19]. The joint focus of the physician and the voice disorders specialist will provide the most comprehensive array of appropriate options for professional voice cases.

References

[1] Heylen L, Wuyts F, Mertens M, et al. Normative voice range profiles of male and female professional voice users. J Voice 2002;16(1):1–7.

[2] Van der Merwe A. Voice dysfunction in the broadcasting professional. Am J Speech Lang Pathol 1995;4:8–10.

[3] Behrman A, Orlikoff R. Instrumentation in voice assessment and treatment: what's the use? Am J Speech Lang Pathol 1997;(6):9–16.

[4] Emerich KA, Titze IR, Švec JG, et al. Vocal range and intensity in actors: a studio versus stage comparison. J Voice 2005;19(1):78–83.

[5] Verdolini K, Titze IR. The application of laboratory formulas to clinical voice management. Am J Speech Lang Pathol 1994;4:62–9.

[6] Nicholosi L, Harryman E, Kresheck J. Terminology of communication disorders: speech-language-hearing. 4th edition. Baltimore (MD): Williams & Wilkins; 1996.

[7] Goldman SL, Hargrave J, Hillman RE, et al. Stress, anxiety, somatic complaints, and voice use in women with vocal nodules: preliminary findings. Am J Speech Lang Pathol 1996;5: 44–54.

[8] Pannbacker M. Voice treatment techniques: a review and recommendations for outcome studies. Am J Speech Lang Pathol 1998;(7):49–64.

[9] Pannbacker M. Treatment of vocal nodules: options and outcomes. Am J Speech Lang Pathol 1999;8:209–17.

[10] Kelchner LN, Horne J, Lee L, et al. Reliability of speech-language pathologist and otolaryngologist ratings of laryngeal signs of reflux in an asymptomatic population using the reflux finding score. J Voice 2006;(Mar):16.

[11] Forrest LA, Weed H. Candida laryngitis appearing as leukoplakia and GERD. J Voice 1998; 12:91–5.

[12] Teachey JC, Kahane JC, Beckford NS. Vocal mechanics in untrained professional singers. J Voice 1991;5(1):51–6.

[13] Shrivastav R, Sapienza CM, Nandur V. Application of psychometric theory to the measurement of voice quality using rating scales. J Speech Lang Hear Res 2005;(48):323–35.

[14] Oates J, Bain B, Davis P, et al. Development of an Auditory–perceptual rating instrument for the operatic singing. J Voice 2006;20(1):71–81.

[15] Jacobson BH, Johnson A, Grywalski C, et al. The voice handicap index (VHI): development and validation. Am J Speech Lang Pathol 1997;6(3):66–70.

[16] Rosen CA, Murry T. Voice handicap index in singers. J Voice 2000;14(3):370–7.

[17] Heman-Ackah YD, Dean CM, Sataloff RT. Strobovideolaryngoscopic findings in singing teachers. J Voice 2002;16(1):81–6.

[18] Blood GW. Efficacy of computer-assisted voice treatment protocol. Am J Speech Lang Pathol 1994;3(1):57.

[19] Timmermans B, De Bodt MS, Wuyts FL, et al. Analysis and evaluation of a voice training program in future professional voice users. J Voice 2005;19(2):202–10.

ELSEVIER
SAUNDERS

Phys Med Rehabil Clin N Am
17 (2006) 761–779

PHYSICAL MEDICINE
AND REHABILITATION
CLINICS OF
NORTH AMERICA

Focal Peripheral Neuropathies in Instrumental Musicians

Richard J. Lederman, MD, PhD

*Department of Neurology and Medical Center for Performing Artists,
Cleveland Clinic Lerner College of Medicine of Case Western Reserve University,
9500 Euclid Avenue, Cleveland, OH 44195, USA*

Peripheral neuropathies may be generalized or focal; the latter may involve a single nerve or even a branch of a particular nerve, or there may be several nerves affected, as in mononeuropathy multiplex. Most focal neuropathies, however, involve only an individual nerve, and generally are characterized as mononeuropathies. The most common cause of a mononeuropathy is compression injury, which may occur at any point along the course of the peripheral nerve. It may be acute or chronic, and may produce either focal loss of myelin or axonal degeneration. The term entrapment neuropathy generally is used to indicate this mechanism, although entrapment usually implies compression at a specific and predictable location where the nerve may be subjected to pressure between body tissues, including bone, ligament, muscle or tendon, blood vessel, or fascial thickening. Compression also may occur from a source outside the body when the nerve lies very superficially, for instance, the ulnar nerve at the elbow or the peroneal nerve at the fibular neck. In most of the literature on peripheral neuropathy, however, the terms entrapment and compression are used interchangeably.

Although entrapment neuropathy is the most common form of focal neuropathy, there are many other causes, including trauma (laceration, contusion), ischemia, tumor, infection, immune-mediated reaction, and physical or chemical injury (eg, radiation, cold, misplaced injections, or local application of toxic substances). This article focuses on the entrapment neuropathies which the author has seen, or that have been reported by others in instrumental musicians.

There is no evidence to suggest that instrumentalists are at higher risk of developing focal neuropathies than anyone else, although there are some specific disorders that appear to be related directly to the playing position

---

E-mail address: ledermr@ccf.org

doi:10.1016/j.pmr.2006.06.009
pmr.theclinics.com

or the manner in which the instrument is held [1]. It is clear, however, that entrapment neuropathies are diagnosed in numerous instrumentalists who seek medical consultation in clinics specializing in performing arts medicine. This, of course, is dependent on the specialty orientation of the clinic and the referral patterns at that particular institution, and on the aggressiveness with which the diagnosis of focal neuropathy is pursued. Entrapment neuropathy was reported in 4% of patients seen at a general musicians' clinic in the United Kingdom [2], in 10% of instrumentalists presenting to an orthopedic hand surgeon interested particularly in musicians' injuries [3], in 11% of those seen at a music medicine clinic in Boston [4], in 19% of instrumentalists presenting to this author (a neurologist), in 22.5% of patients treated at a musicians' clinic under the direction of a hand surgeon at the Mayo Clinic [5], and in 48% of instrumentalists referred to a neurologist with a special interest in peripheral nerve disorders [6].

Specific focal neuropathies in instrumentalists

Table 1 lists the mononeuropathies that are discussed in this section. This represents the frequency in patients seen in the author's performing artists' clinic, and it should not be construed as the actual prevalence of these disorders among instrumentalists in general.

The distribution of symptoms and signs in all the neuromuscular disorders, including focal neuropathies, of instrumentalists seen in the author's clinic tend to show instrument-specific patterns, as demonstrated in Table 2. Violinists and violists, particularly, have a predominance of left arm problems, whereas keyboard players are more likely to have problems with the right arm and hand. Oboists and clarinetists, among the woodwind players, more commonly have pain and sensorimotor symptoms in the right hand and arm, probably because this is the weight-bearing hand, whereas brass

Table 1
Mononeuropathies in instrumental musicians (author's series)

Nerve/syndrome	Number of patients
Thoracic outlet syndrome	76
Ulnar neuropathy (elbow)	73
Carpal tunnel syndrome (CTS)	66
Cervical radiculopathy	36
Cranial neuropathy	18
Digital neuropathy	17
Median nerve, non-CTS	12
Ulnar neuropathy, not at elbow	8
Long thoracic neuropathy	7
Radial neuropathy	6
Lumbar radiculopathy	6
Other	17
Total	342

Table 2
Upper extremity affected in instrumentalists (%)

Instrument Group	R	L	Bilateral		
			R>	=	<L
Strings, bowed	25	55	4	10	6
Strings, plucked	27	43	4	17	9
Keyboard	43	24	11	14	8
Woodwind	44	23	9	17	7
Brass	27	45	6	12	9
Percussion	34	18	0	39	8

players are more likely to have symptoms on the left, although limb problems are relatively infrequent. Drummers tend to have bilateral symptoms.

Thoracic outlet syndrome

The most common focal neuropathy in the author's series is also the most controversial. The issues regarding this diagnosis are recognized and have been discussed extensively in the literature [7–10]. Thoracic outlet syndrome (TOS) in musicians has been reported by others. A young flutist was among the patients with the pain and paresthesias form of TOS described by Lascelles and colleagues [11]. Charness [6] diagnosed TOS in 40 of 117 instrumental musicians in his series with nerve entrapment. Hochberg [4] reported 70 cases of TOS out of the total of 1000 musicians seen at his clinic, and Winspur [2] diagnosed nine with TOS out of 137 musicians with "specific orthopaedic/rheumatological" conditions. The author's series includes 76 instrumentalists, none of whom had the true neurogenic form of TOS.

The diagnosis of the common symptomatic or nonspecific form of TOS is based on criteria that have not been validated formally. The criteria the author used included:

- Pain, most often in the forearm, ulnar side more than radial, but sometimes more proximally in the upper arm or shoulder or more distally in the hand.
- Sensory symptoms, including numbness, tingling, burning, or swelling, again in the same distribution as the pain.
- Symptoms generally associated with specific positions or activities, at least initially, but they may become more constant over time.
- Symptoms can be provoked by specific maneuvers such as downward traction on the arm, hyperabduction of the arm at the shoulder, or cervical rotation and flexion [12].
- Normal neurologic examination with no significant motor, sensory, or reflex abnormality [13].

The patients in the author's series met at least four of these five criteria.

Of the 76 patients with TOS, 56 were women, and 20 were men. Age at evaluation ranged from 15 to 47 years, with a mean of 25 years. There were 34 bowed string players, including 26 violinists or violists, seven cellists, and one double bassist; 19 keyboard players; and 13 woodwind instrumentalists, including nine flutists. Among the string players, 31 had unilateral involvement. Twenty-two had left arm involvement, and nine had right arm involvement. Keyboard players were more likely to have bilateral symptoms (eight), with six having left and five right arm involvement only. Symptoms in the flute players were divided evenly between right and left. About half the 76 patients had what has been called the droopy shoulder configuration [14] (Fig. 1).

Ulnar neuropathy

The next most commonly diagnosed disorder was ulnar neuropathy at the elbow. There were 73 musicians identified with this disorder, 38 men and 35 women. They ranged in age from 15 to 71 years at the time of evaluation (mean, 39 years). Of the 23 keyboard players with ulnar neuropathy at the elbow, 14 had only left arm symptoms; four had right arm symptoms only, and five had bilateral involvement. Among all the string players so diagnosed (36), 34 had left arm involvement, and five had right (three were bilateral). If one looks at only the bowed string players, the findings are even more striking. Of 28 instrumentalists, including 13 violinists, eight violists, four cellists, and three double bass players, 25 had left arm/hand symptoms, and three had bilateral complaints; no one had just right hand numbness. If one considers the playing position for these instruments (Fig. 2), there appears to be important information relating to the pathogenesis of the symptoms. The left elbow is maintained in a flexed position, combined with supination, at least in the violinists and violists, and accompanied by repetitive flexion and extension of the digits, whereas the right elbow is flexed and extended repeatedly with bowing. This suggests that sustained flexion at the elbow, with the addition of accompanying repeated finger movement, may be much more likely to produce ulnar neuropathy than repeated flexion and extension of the elbow (which also has been suggested as a causative

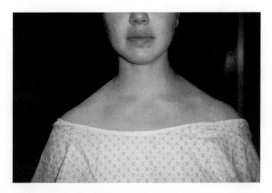

Fig. 1. Droopy shoulder configuration in a patient with thoracic outlet syndrome. Note the relatively long neck and the sloping shoulders.

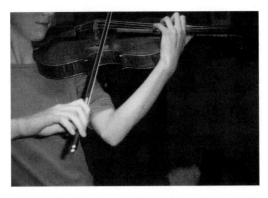

Fig. 2. Ulnar neuropathy at the elbow in a violinist's left arm. Note playing position with sustained elbow flexion and forearm supination.

mechanism [15]). Keyboard players also had left ulnar neuropathy more frequently, which may be a bit more difficult to explain. It might be suggested that, because the right hand carries the melody line and is more likely to range widely on the keyboard, this may translate into more sustained left elbow flexion and more dynamic elbow movement on the right. The situation may, then, be similar to what is experienced by the string players. Among 12 woodwind instrumentalists, for whom the playing position of the elbows is both more static and more symmetrical (if anything, the left elbow is more flexed than the right), eight patients had right-sided symptoms, and six had left hand involvement (two had bilateral involvement).

Charness [6] found 72 examples of ulnar neuropathy at the elbow among the 192 nerve entrapment syndromes identified in 117 instrumentalists. He also found a predominance of left-sided symptoms in the string players, with right-sided or bilateral involvement among pianists. Hochberg [4] reported 40 cases of ulnar neuropathy in the 1000 musicians evaluated in their clinic.

Carpal tunnel syndrome

Although carpal tunnel syndrome (CTS) is the most common upper extremity nerve entrapment in the general population, it has been slightly less frequent among instrumentalists in the author's series, as it was in Charness' series [6]. Amadio and Russotti [5] reported five cases of CTS among 40 musicians evaluated (13%). Winspur [2] found four patients who had CTS among 323 musicians seen (1%), and Dawson [16], a hand surgeon, reviewed 98 cases of CTS from a series of 1354 instrumental musicians seen in his practice (7%). Charness [6] identified 24 patients who had CTS (12 bilateral) out of the 117 instrumentalists with entrapment neuropathies (21%).

Among the 66 musicians in the author's series with CTS, 40 were women, and 26 were men. They ranged in age from 17 to 79 years at the time of evaluation, with a mean of 44 years. Keyboard players comprised the single largest group, including 19 pianists, eight organists, and two accordion players. Seventeen had bilateral involvement. Eight had right side involvement only, and four had left side involvement only. Twenty-seven of the 29 keyboard musicians were right-handed. Among the 13 violinists and violists, nine had right greater than left or right hand involvement only, and four had left hand symptoms only. All but one was right-handed. Again, there is no evidence to suggest that instrumentalists are more prone to develop CTS than others, nor is there evidence that the playing position is particularly likely to predispose to the development of CTS. The gender distribution, age range, and symptom description are similar to what is seen in the general population [17].

Cervical radiculopathy

Instrumentalists with cervical radiculopathy had the characteristic clinical syndrome of neck pain, with spread to the interscapular region and upper extremity, along with sensory symptoms with or without motor and reflex impairment, depending on the specific root involved.

Few reports of cervical root lesions in instrumentalists are available. Blau and Henson [18] described three (possibly four) musicians with radiculopathy, including two bowed string players (possibly a third). Bejjani and colleagues [19,20] reported a harpist with a left C6 radiculopathy, attributed to asymmetric neck position related to playing. The present series includes 36 instrumentalists, 27 men and nine women. As might be expected, the average age of 50 years was older than that seen in other nerve entrapment disorders, with a range at evaluation of 29 years up to age 90. It has been suggested that the playing position of violinists (and violists) predisposes to the development of cervical radiculopathy [21]. Although this may seem intuitively likely, the author cannot confirm this from his clinical experience. Of the 499 violinists/violists seen, only 11 (2%) have been diagnosed with a cervical radiculopathy; furthermore, less than one third of the total group with this diagnosis have been violinists or violists. It has been suggested [21] that violinists are particularly likely to have left-sided involvement and pianists right-sided symptoms. Among the violinists and violists in this series, four had right, six left, and one bilateral cervical radiculopathies; among keyboard players, seven had left; two had right, and one had bilateral involvement. Although the series is small, it does not strongly support a significant tendency toward lateralization, compared, for instance, with the tendency regarding ulnar neuropathy among the bowed string players. With respect to the cervical root affected among the entire group of 36, one had C5 involvement; 15, C6; 11, C7; and 7, C8. Two were indeterminate.

Cranial neuropathies

Focal disorders of cranial nerves are an infrequent cause of problems with performance. The most common in the author's series of 18 patients was the occurrence of localized sensory (and sometimes motor) impairment of the lip, primarily among brass instrumentalists. Martin and Lederman [22] reported a case in a trumpeter, and the author has seen eight of these, seven in brass players (Fig. 3) and one in a clarinetist. The usual explanation is localized excessive pressure on the lip from the mouthpiece externally against the dental ridge underlying the affected lip segment. A similar case was described by Frucht [23]. Also included in the author's series are three musicians with traumatic injury to branches of the trigeminal or facial nerve (two from dental surgery) and two cases of Bell's palsy, both severely affecting playing (French horn and clarinet; Fig. 4).

Digital neuropathy

Seventeen instrumentalists in the author's series had focal involvement of a digital nerve; 11 were playing-related. The most common was flutists' neuropathy, first described by Cynamon [24]; this involves the radial aspect of the left index finger, caused by excessive pressure on the instrument. A similar mechanism was suspected in a violinist, a cellist, and two guitarists, all thought to be related to pressure of the index finger against the edge of the fingerboard. An unusual example of a digital neuropathy is seen in Fig. 5. This marimba player was practicing for hours at a time with four mallets and developed focal numbness of the left middle finger. All of these have resolved with reduction in playing and technical changes. Six of the digital neuropathies were unrelated to the playing the instrument, although significantly impacting the ability to play. This group includes one young Asian pianist who played so much ping-pong that he developed numbness of the right middle finger from pressure on the paddle. Patrone and colleagues [25] described a young violinist with digital nerve compression involving the small finger of the left hand, associated with joint hypermobility.

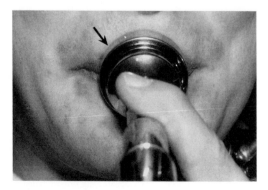

Fig. 3. Sensory loss involving the right upper lip of a trombonist. The arrow points to the presumed site of compression of the mouthpiece against the upper lip.

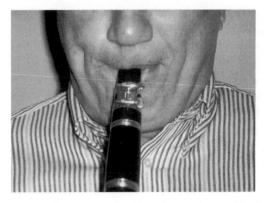

Fig. 4. Bell's palsy on the left in a clarinetist. Note the asymmetry of lip function; there was leakage of air on the left as he played.

Other focal neuropathies

Not all median neuropathies are associated with CTS. Several patients in the author's series had traumatic injury to the median nerve in the forearm or hand from surgery, venous or arterial puncture, or fractures. A subgroup of four patients had anterior interosseous neuropathies [26] with weakness of flexion of the tip of the thumb and index finger, primarily. At least three of these were thought to represent examples of neuralgic amyotrophy, and complete or nearly full resolution was seen in all four patients. Median neuropathy in the upper forearm occurs in the pronator syndrome, first described in a pianist by Kopell and Thompson [27]. One of the patients reported by Morris and Peter [28] was a fiddler, and Charness [6] described a cellist with proximal median neuropathy; this patient was said also to have TOS and an ulnar neuropathy at the elbow. A harpist in the author's series developed

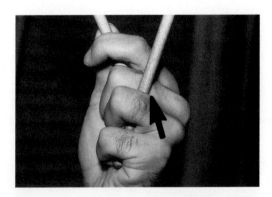

Fig. 5. Digital nerve compression (ulnar aspect of left long finger), caused by prolonged four-mallet playing of the marimba. There was sensory loss distal to the point of compression (*arrow*).

a pronator syndrome after having to tune several harps repeatedly for a concert [29]. She recovered fully over many months.

Ulnar neuropathy at sites other than the elbow is much less common. Wainapel and Cole [30] described two flutists with ulnar entrapment at Guyon's canal at the wrist, presenting with pure sensory or pure motor symptoms. The author's series included three cases of distal ulnar neuropathy. One was a professional violinist who compressed the right ulnar nerve in the hand while participating in a biking marathon, covering over 750 miles in 3 days. He also had a median neuropathy at the wrist on the left. Fortunately, both deficits recovered fully over a few months. Other types of trauma accounted for four additional cases.

The author previously reported five cases of unilateral long thoracic neuropathy [31], causing shoulder pain and a winged scapula. Two subsequent cases have been seen in the author's clinic. Five involved the right side, and two involved the left. At least five of these were thought to represent examples of neuralgic amyotrophy; two were of uncertain cause, possibly traumatic. Again, partial if not complete recovery can be expected, but pain and shoulder dysfunction can persist for many months.

Radial mononeuropathy has been uncommon in the author's series. The author has seen two patients with proximal injury in the upper arm, one from trauma and another from use of a crutch. There are also two cases of radial cutaneous branch injury. Posterior interosseous neuropathy in a musician was reported by Woltman and Learmonth [32] in their classic paper describing five cases. Charness [6] reported seven such cases in musicians. The author's series included only one patient, and he was seen only after having undergone radial tunnel decompression. Maffulli and Maffulli [33] reported transient posterior interosseous nerve entrapment in 11 violinists. Their initial report indicated involvement of the left arm and attributed the compression to prolonged pronation of the forearm with playing. When it was pointed out that the left forearm is supinated during playing [34], the authors indicated that they had meant to indicate involvement of the right arm. The author has not seen a single case of this in over 500 violinists and violists personally evaluated.

Lumbosacral radiculopathy is a common problem in the general population and is not likely to occur less frequently in musicians. It may not have a direct impact on the ability to play, however, and hence it was seen relatively infrequently in this series. Of the six cases included, two were in organists, and this did have a significant effect on their ability to use the foot pedals.

Diagnostic approach to the instrumentalist with focal neuropathies

The musician being seen in medical consultation for a playing-related problem is, first and foremost, a patient seeking help, and, as such, he or she is entitled to what would be done for any patient. That means beginning with a thorough history and as complete an examination as seems warranted for the problem being analyzed. The history of necessity should include an inquiry into the specific symptoms, eliciting whatever information is needed to understand the problem. In the case of a musician, it is important to determine the relationship between the symptoms and the instrumentalist's activities, both musical and nonmusical. It is critical, therefore, to inquire about practice habits and playing technique. Has the onset coincided with a change in practice time, preparation for a concert or audition, new instrument, change in teacher, attempt to modify technique, learning a particularly difficult new piece, or change in position in the orchestra (eg, inside versus outside chair)? Has there been some change in nonmusical activities (a new job to help make ends meet, a different athletic activity) or an added social or psychological stress?

The physical examination should focus primarily on the musculoskeletal and neurological systems. It also should use the techniques known to be helpful for the suspected nerve entrapment (eg, the Tinel, Phalen, or carpal compression test for CTS; the elbow flexion test for ulnar neuropathy; the Spurling maneuver for cervical radiculopathy; resistive forearm supination or resistive middle finger extension for the radial tunnel syndrome; or one of the several provocative maneuvers said to facilitate the diagnosis of TOS) [35].

Because the symptoms presumably relate in some way to the playing of the instrument, whether caused by playing, or, perhaps more commonly, having an impact on the ability to play, physicians who see musicians frequently have emphasized the need to watch them play as part of the diagnostic analysis. If at all feasible, they should be advised to bring their instrument(s) to the appointment, and part of the time should be spent observing them as they play. Obviously, pianists and organists cannot bring their instrument, but many physicians who see musicians regularly should have ready access to a piano or alternate keyboard. For those traveling long distances, it can be equally difficult to come with a harp or double bass, but often one can arrange to borrow an instrument from a local musician. Physicians often are asked how useful this can be, when they cannot provide expert opinions on technical aspects of all instrumental performance, if any at all. What one can recognize, however, are postures or positions that may predispose to nerve entrapment at some site (eg, excessive wrist flexion or unusual neck or upper trunk position). One has to be extremely careful, however, not to assume that any particular playing position is necessarily wrong or improper. The history of music is replete with unorthodox practices that had no apparent deleterious effects on the instrumentalist and, in fact, were critical to his or her success (think, for instance, of Dizzy Gillespie's puffed-out cheeks).

The usefulness of ancillary studies is also not different, basically, for the musician with suspected nerve entrapment. Whether one looks for underlying systemic or metabolic disease depends on the specific situation. Imaging studies for some focal nerve compression syndromes, such as cervical or lumbar MR imaging for radiculopathy, will be employed more commonly than for most others. There has been increasing enthusiasm, however, for MR imaging in more peripheral nerve lesions also [36]. Radiographs of the elbow may be useful for diagnosing ulnar neuropathy in musicians and others, as has been emphasized by Amadio [37] and by Nolan and Eaton [38]. Recent interest in ultrasonography for evaluating CTS [39, 40] and ulnar neuropathy [41] and other focal nerve entrapments, also has emerged.

Electrodiagnostic (EDX) studies are most likely to be helpful and justifiable. Musicians, if anything, may be a bit more reluctant to agree to electromyography (EMG) than most patients. Generally, however, they are willing to proceed when the rationale and safety are adequately explained.

The approach to EDX studies can differ widely from one laboratory to another. Practice parameters have been published by professional societies for CTS [42] and ulnar neuropathy [43], although it must be recognized that these are constructs by a committee and individual laboratories may have areas of disagreement. MacLean [44] has discussed the EDX approach to CTS and ulnar neuropathy in the instrumentalist. The minimum requirements for investigation of CTS include median sensory nerve conduction studies across the wrist, with comparison with an ulnar or radial sensory study. Most also would include a median motor study. Confirmation that there is focal slowing at the wrist requires comparison with a segment proximally or distally. Various additional conduction studies may be helpful if the standard procedures are normal or equivocal. At least a minimal screening needle EMG is performed routinely in the author's laboratory, even if the nerve conduction studies are convincing, but this is not considered mandatory by some others.

In the author's series, 56 of the 66 patients diagnosed with CTS underwent EDX studies, and 53 had abnormal results (95%), bilaterally in 37 of the 53 (70%). EDX studies in patients who have ulnar neuropathy are less likely to be helpful. About two thirds of the author's patients diagnosed with ulnar neuropathy, based on characteristic symptoms, and, less commonly, convincing neurological signs, underwent EDX studies. Roughly half of those had focal slowing in the region of the elbow, and fewer had evidence of axon loss. Charness and colleagues [45] studied 27 musicians who had clinically diagnosed ulnar neuropathy. Of 17 studied with surface recording, only five (29%) showed focal slowing at the elbow. Using near-nerve recording, 15 of 19 (79%) showed reduced conduction velocity. The technical difficulties in doing these studies, and the time required, make this relatively impractical in most medical centers. MacLean [44] emphasized the importance of localizing the point of compression to the ulnar groove or the cubital tunnel (much of the literature fails to differentiate these and lumps them together, incorrectly) by using needle stimulation. Additional discussions of the controversies involved in confirming and localizing ulnar neuropathy electrodiagnostically are available elsewhere [46].

EDX studies in cervical radiculopathy can be helpful in confirming the localization and identifying the presence of axonal injury, which may influence the decision to consider a more aggressive and invasive approach to treatment. Of the 36 musicians in this series, 18 underwent EDX studies (50%), and 15 showed evidence of axon loss, mostly chronic rather than active or ongoing; one additional study was considered equivocal. Denervation was seen in C6 distribution in five patients. It was seen in C7 distribution in five cases, and in C8 distribution in six cases, one with additional contralateral C7 changes.

The usefulness of various EDX studies in TOS has been debated. The author has studied relatively few of his musician patients, roughly one third, primarily to exclude an alternative diagnosis. The author has not found any specific abnormalities in these patients, a finding similar to the experiences of most investigators who have studied musicians (and others) who have TOS [2,6,47–50].

Treatment of focal neuropathies

The approach to treating nerve compression syndromes in musicians is, in many ways, similar to that advocated for any other patient. The approach depends on many factors, including the desires and expectations of that patient [51]. Musicians as a group tend to be very reluctant to consider any of the invasive approaches, not just surgery, but injections and even oral medications. At the same time, however, they are often extremely anxious to obtain a quick fix, to the point of requesting that something be done today to get them back to playing tomorrow. Another particular feature of treatment of the instrumentalist is related to the extraordinary level of neuromuscular control that is required to play at a high level. A musician may note a subtle degree of impairment associated with relatively mild nerve entrapment that someone with lesser neuromuscular demands would not be aware of or might be willing to accept. This may result in the demand to do something more aggressive, such as surgery, when the clinical or, perhaps, electrical abnormality seems modest to the physician.

Box 1 lists numerous treatment approaches that may be considered, either alone or in various combinations. Reduction in playing time or a decrease in the duration of each practice segment may be sufficient, in some cases, to alleviate the symptoms. Usually, however, this would be accompanied by other changes, such as modifying playing position or altering technique. An example might be the brass player's sensory loss on the lip, which might resolve with some time off or reduced playing, although it likely would be combined with instruction in decreasing the tendency to pull the mouthpiece tightly against the lip or altering slightly the angle at which the instrument is held. Similarly, Bell's palsy in a wind player likely will have to await the resolution over time, although initial treatment with antiviral therapy and perhaps oral steroids should be considered, if the musician is seen early enough. One of the author's patients, a French horn player, was able to resume playing before complete recovery had taken place by moving

---

Box 1. Treatment modalities for focal neuropathies

General measures
Modification of:
- Practice schedule/playing time
- Posture/playing position
- Technique
- Instrument

Stress management/tension reduction
Medication (analgesics, anti-inflammatory)

Specific measures
Therapeutic exercises
Splints/orthoses
Local corticosteroid injection
Surgery

---

the mouthpiece slightly toward the unaffected side and taping the affected lips together to reduce air leak. The digital neuropathy of flutists may subside with decreased playing, but this should be accompanied by a reduction in the pressure being exerted by the left index finger against the barrel of the instrument. The latter can be modified further by an adaptive device to diffuse that pressure [52].

Symptoms of CTS can be alleviated by decreased hand activity, but a change in the wrist position, with even slightly less flexion while playing (Fig. 6), may reduce the symptoms more rapidly, and, more importantly, help ensure that they not recur when a full playing schedule is resumed. Wearing a wrist splint at night can help to diminish daytime symptoms of

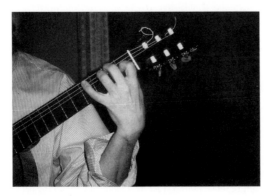

Fig. 6. Pronounced left wrist flexion in a guitarist with carpal tunnel syndrome on the left.

CTS, and prevent the nocturnal awakening so characteristic of the syndrome. Wearing an elbow splint or sleeve at night to prevent excessive flexion can help reduce symptoms of ulnar neuropathy, although it usually will be combined with behavioral modification such as avoiding leaning on the elbows and trying to decrease the degree and time of elbow flexion during daytime activities, including playing.

Modification of playing posture is an integral component treating TOS, along with more specific therapeutic exercises. Instrument modification can be very helpful in reducing the stresses that predispose to focal neuropathies. Norris [53,54] has been particularly innovative in this regard. Cervical radiculopathy in a violinist or violist can be helped by decreasing the required neck flexion required to hold the instrument, especially in those players with longer necks. A specially designed chin rest (Fig. 7) was career-saving for a violinist in the author's practice, whose radicular symptoms were markedly reduced with this adaptation.

Other general measures for treating focal neuropathies may include various techniques for reducing muscular tension and stress, which often contribute to the symptoms or indeed to the pathogenesis of the nerve compression. Relaxation techniques such as yoga, meditation, and biofeedback, and body awareness techniques such as those from Alexander and Feldenkrais can make a significant difference in the recovery from nerve compression symptoms and prevention of recurrence.

Specific therapeutic exercise regimens have been suggested for several focal neuropathies, most notably, TOS. Initially suggested by Peet and colleagues [55], who first used the term thoracic outlet syndrome, various nonsurgical therapeutic approaches have been suggested [56–58]. Virtually all, however, are intended to modify the anatomic configuration of the upper trunk between the neck and shoulder. Other nerve entrapments also can be treated with physical therapy, designed to mobilize the affected nerve

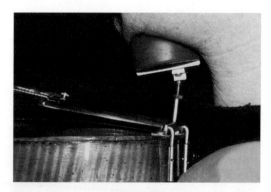

Fig. 7. Customized adjustable chin rest used by a violinist with a long neck (he is 6 ft 4 in) and chronic cervical radiculopathy.

(eg, gliding techniques) and reduce the likelihood of tense muscles exerting pressure on adjacent nerves.

Injection of corticosteroids has been one of the standard approaches to focal neuropathies, particularly CTS [59,60]. Most authors seem to agree that it can be safe and effective, but it is generally a short-term solution, unless hand activity can be modified to prevent recurrence [61]. Cervical or lumbar epidural injection of corticosteroids also can be helpful in alleviating the symptoms of spinal radiculopathy, again usually temporarily, but often this is sufficient to allow the underlying disc protrusion or root swelling to subside on its own.

The literature concerning surgical decompression for nerve entrapment is too vast to consider reviewing here. Numerous reviews focusing on musicians are available [3,37,38,62,63]. Discussion of specific techniques (eg, open versus endoscopic surgery for CTS or simple decompression of the ulnar nerve at the elbow versus transposition with subcutaneous or submuscular implantation) is beyond the scope of this article. The issue of surgical management of TOS also has been the subject of intense and often vitriolic debate. Most reviews have emphasized the desirability of an initial conservative approach, although Roos [64] downplayed the overall usefulness, at least in moderate-to-severe cases. It is safe to state, however, that most physicians involved in performing arts medicine would consider surgery a last resort after all other therapeutic modalities have failed [65]. There appear to be major regional differences in approach. Surgery for TOS seems to be far more common in the United States than, for instance, in the United Kingdom. Even within the United States, surgery may be used much more frequently in some centers than in others [7]. The specific surgical approach also varies, with some favoring the transaxillary procedure popularized by Roos [66]. Others prefer a supraclavicular approach, and some use a combined procedure [67]. The localization of symptoms may influence the choice; suspected involvement of the lower plexus tends to favor the transaxillary approach. Critics of surgical management, including those who do not even accept the diagnosis, have emphasized the potential complications [68,69].

Treatment outcome

Data regarding outcome of treatment for focal neuropathies in musicians is sparse. The author first reported results in 1989 [29], looking at 65 instrumentalists with various nerve entrapments, mostly TOS, at 1 to 10 years after treatment. Of these, 74% had a good or excellent outcome, the former indicating at most mild and intermittent symptoms. Nine (14%) had equivocal improvement, and eight (12%) had a poor outcome, including four who had no treatment recommended. These data have been updated periodically, although not comprehensively [13]. About 75% of patients who have TOS have a favorable outcome, including the only two in the author's series treated surgically. Of the author's patients who have CTS, about half ultimately opt for surgical treatment, usually after extended conservative therapy. The results of carpal tunnel release (CTR) have been very favorable, with about 90% reporting complete or nearly full recovery. Some of those choosing to defer CTR continue to be symptomatic and may have had to modify their playing schedules.

Among the author's patients with ulnar neuropathy, most are treated nonsurgically, and most are able to continue playing, with manageable symptoms. The author is aware of 13 who have undergone surgical treatment; two others have been offered surgery and may have had it elsewhere. Of the 13, nine have had a good outcome and are back to full-time playing. Follow-up information is unavailable in one additional musician. One woman, an organist, has had some residual ulnar symptoms following surgery, but also had severe pain at the tip of the small finger. The author suspected a glomus tumor and, indeed, this was documented with MR imaging. She has had an excellent result from removal of this lesion. Currently, only five of the 36 patients with cervical radiculopathy have required decompressive surgery, and all have done well. The remaining instrumentalists have had adequate relief with conservative measures.

In the only other long-term study of musicians with entrapment neuropathies, Dawson reported a series of 98 instrumentalists who had CTS [16]. Of 57 managed nonsurgically, 27 had at least moderate improvement, but another 27 had no follow-up. Of 38 patients treated surgically (total of 50 hands), all did well, although one patient had a subsequent recurrence.

Summary

Instrumental musicians often seek medical consultation for symptoms suggestive of nerve entrapment. About 20% of those seen in the author's performing artists' clinic were diagnosed with a focal neuropathy. In general, neuropathies that are most common in the overall population tend also to be most common among musicians, although some exceptions exist, including, for example, localized peri–oral sensory syndromes associated with playing a brass instrument, and, possibly, ulnar neuropathies related to the playing position of bowed string players. The diagnosis is made, as always, by careful clinical assessment, including observation of the instrumentalist playing, with ancillary procedures such as nerve conduction studies and needle electromyography adding to the accuracy of the diagnosis. Treatment is similar to that used in nonmusicians, but certain factors, including the musician's requirement for extraordinary neuromuscular dexterity, may influence the therapeutic decisions. Very limited long-term outcome results are available, and additional studies in musicians would be helpful in determining the most appropriate therapeutic approaches. Virtually no longitudinal studies have been performed to look at methods for preventing these disorders.

References

[1] Dawson DM, Hallett M, Wilbourn AJ. Nerve entrapments in musicians. In: Dawson DM, Hallett M, Wilbourn AJ, editors. Entrapment neuropathies. 3rd edition. Philadelphia: Lippincott-Raven; 1999. p. 443–50.

[2] Winspur I, Wynn Parry CB. The musician's hand. J Hand Surg 1997;22B:433–40.

[3] Dawson WJ. Experience with hand and upper-extremity problems in 1000 instrumentalists. Med Probl Perform Art 1995;10:128–33.

[4] Hochberg FH, Lederman RJ. Upper extremity difficulties of musicians. In: Hunter JM, Mackin EJ, Callahan AD, editors. Rehabilitation of the hand: surgery and therapy. 4th edition. St. Louis (MO): Mosby; 1995. p. 1795–808.

[5] Amadio PC, Russotti GM. Evaluation and treatment of hand and wrist disorders in musicians. Hand Clin 1990;6:405–16.

[6] Charness ME. Unique upper extremity disorders in musicians. In: Millender LH, Louis DS, Simmons BP, editors. Occupational disorders of the upper extremity. New York: Churchill Livingstone; 1992. p. 227–52.

[7] Lederman RJ. Thoracic outlet syndrome: review of the controversies and a report of 17 instrumental musicians. Med Probl Perform Art 1987;2:87–91.

[8] Roos DB. The thoracic outlet syndrome is underrated. Arch Neurol 1990;47:327–8.

[9] Wilbourn AJ. The thoracic outlet syndrome is overdiagnosed. Arch Neurol 1990;47: 328–30.

[10] Hachinski V. The thoracic outlet syndrome. Arch Neurol 1990;47:330.

[11] Lascelles RG, Mohr PD, Neary D, et al. The thoracic outlet syndrome. Brain 1977;100: 601–12.

[12] Lindgren KA, Leino E, Manninen H. Cervical rotation lateral flexion test in brachialgia. Arch Phys Med Rehabil 1992;73:735–7.

[13] Lederman RJ. Neuromuscular and musculoskeletal problems in instrumental musicians. Muscle Nerve 2003;27:549–61.

[14] Swift TR, Nichols FT. The droopy shoulder syndrome. Neurology 1984;34:212–5.

[15] Stewart JD. Focal peripheral neuropathies, 3rd edition. Philadelphia: Lippincott Williams & Wilkins; 1999. p. 251.

[16] Dawson WJ. Carpal tunnel syndrome in instrumentalists: a review of 15 years' experience. Med Probl Perform Art 1999;14:25–9.

[17] Rosenbaum RB, Ochoa JL. Carpal tunnel syndrome and other disorder of the median nerve. 2nd edition. Boston: Butterworth-Heinemann; 2002. p. 31–54.

[18] Blau JN, Henson RA. Neurological disorders in performing musicians. In: Critchley M, Henson RA, editors. Music and the brain: studies in the neurology of music. London: Heinemann; 1977. p. 301–22.

[19] Bejjani FJ, Kaye GM, Benham M. Musculoskeletal and neuromuscular conditions of instrumental musicians. Arch Phys Med Rehabil 1996;77:406–13.

[20] Bejjani FJ, Kaye GM, Cheu JW. Performing artists' occupational disorders and related therapies. In: DeLisa JA, Gans BM, editors. Rehabilitation medicine: principles and practice. 3rd edition. Philadelphia: Lippincott-Raven; 1998. p. 1627–59.

[21] Rozmaryn LM. Upper extremity disorders in performing artists. Md Med J 1993;42: 255–60.

[22] Martin WE, Lederman RJ. Trumpet player's neuropathy. JAMA 1987;257:1526.

[23] Frucht S. Anterior superior alveolar neuropathy: an occupational neuropathy of the embouchure. J Neurol Neurosurg Psychiatry 2000;69:562–7.

[24] Cynamon KB. Flutist's neuropathy. N Engl J Med 1981;305:961.

[25] Patrone NA, Hoppman RA, Whaley J, Schmidt R. Digital nerve compression in a violinist with benign hypermobility: a case study. Med Probl Perform Art 1989;4:91–4.

[26] Lederman RJ. Anterior interosseous neuropathy in instrumental musicians. Med Probl Perform Art 2006;21:137–41.

[27] Kopell HP, Thompson WAL. Pronator syndrome: a confirmed case and its diagnosis. N Engl J Med 1958;259:713–5.

[28] Morris HH, Peters BH. Pronator syndrome: clinical and electrophysiological features in seven cases. J Neurol Neurosurg Psychiatry 1976;39:461–4.

[29] Lederman RJ. Peripheral nerve disorders in instrumentalists. Ann Neurol 1989;26:640–6.

[30] Wainapel SF, Cole JL. The not-so-magic flute: two cases of distal ulnar nerve entrapment. Med Probl Perform Art 1988;3:63–5.

[31] Lederman RJ. Long thoracic neuropathy in instrumental musicians: an often unrecognized cause of shoulder pain. Med Probl Perform Art 1996;11:116–9.

[32] Woltman HW, Learmonth JR. Progressive paralysis of the nervus interosseus dorsalis. Brain 1934;57:25–31.

[33] Maffulli N, Maffulli F. Transient entrapment neuropathy of the posterior interosseous nerve in violin players. J Neurol Neurosurg Psychiatry 1991;54:65–7.

[34] Lederman RJ. Transient entrapment neuropathy of the posterior interosseous nerve in violin players. J Neurol Neurosurg Psychiatry 1991;54:1031.

[35] Atasoy E. Thoracic outlet compression syndrome. Orthop Clin N Am 1996;27:265–303.

[36] Grant GA, Britz GW, Goodkin R, et al. The utility of magnetic resonance imaging in evaluating peripheral nerve disorders. Muscle Nerve 2002;25:314–31.

[37] Amadio PC. Diagnosis and treatment of ulnar nerve entrapment at the elbow and carpal tunnel syndrome in musicians. Med Probl Perform Art 1993;8:53–9.

[38] Nolan WB, Eaton RG. Evaluation and treatment of cubital tunnel syndrome in musicians. Med Probl Perform Art 1993;8:47–51.

[39] Beekman R, Visser LH. Sonography in the diagnosis of carpal tunnel syndrome: a critical review of the literature. Muscle Nerve 2003;27:26–33.

[40] Kele H, Verheggen R, Bitterman HJ, et al. The potential value of ultrasonography in the evaluation of carpal tunnel syndrome. Neurology 2003;61:389–91.

[41] Beekman R, van der Plas JPL, Uitdehaag BMJ, et al. Clinical, electrodiagnostic, and sonographic studies in ulnar neuropathy at the elbow. Muscle Nerve 2004;30:202–8.

[42] American Association of Electrodiagnostic Medicine, American Academy of Neurology, American Academy of Physical Medicine and Rehabilitation. Practice parameter for electrodiagnostic studies in carpal tunnel syndrome: summary statement. Muscle Nerve 2002;25: 918–22.

[43] American Association of Electrodiagnostic Medicine, American Academy of Neurology, American Academy of Physical Medicine and Rehabilitation. Practice parameter for electrodiagnostic studies in ulnar neuropathy at the elbow: summary statement. Muscle Nerve 1999;22:408–11.

[44] MacLean IC. Carpal tunnel syndrome and cubital tunnel syndrome: the electrodiagnostic viewpoint. Med Probl Perform Art 1993;8:41–5.

[45] Charness ME, Ross MH, Shefner JM. Ulnar neuropathy and dystonic flexion of the fourth and fifth digits: clinical correlation in musicians. Muscle Nerve 1996;19:431–7.

[46] Campbell WW, Greenberg MK, Krendel DA, et al. The electrodiagnostic evaluation of patients with ulnar neuropathy at the elbow: literature review of the usefulness of nerve conduction studies and electromyography. Muscle Nerve 1999;22(Suppl 8):S175–205.

[47] Daube JR. Nerve conduction studies in the thoracic outlet syndrome. Neurology 1975;23:347.

[48] Newmark J, Levy SR, Hochberg FH. Somatosensory evoked potentials in thoracic outlet syndrome. Arch Neurol 1985;42:1036.

[49] Veilleux M, Stevens JC, Campbell JK. Somatosensory evoked potentials: lack of value for diagnosis of thoracic outlet syndrome. Muscle Nerve 1988;11:571–5.

[50] Wilbourn AJ, Porter JM. Thoracic outlet syndromes. Spine. State of the Art Reviews 1988;2: 597–626.

[51] Dommerholt J, Norris RN, Shaheen M. Therapeutic management of the instrumental musician. In: Sataloff RT, Brandfonbrener AG, Lederman RJ, editors. Performing arts medicine. 2nd edition. San Diego (CA): Singular; 1998. p. 277–90.

[52] Andersen JI. Orthotic device for flutist's digital nerve compression. Med Probl Perform Art 1990;5:91–3.

[53] Norris RN, Dommerholt J. Applied ergonomics: adaptive equipment and instrument modification for musicians. In: Sataloff RT, Brandfonbrener AG, Lederman RJ, editors. Performing arts medicine. 2nd edition. San Diego (CA): Singular; 1998. p. 261–75.

[54] Norris RN. Applied ergonomics. In: Tubiana R, Amadio PC, editors. Medical problems of the instrumentalist musician. London: Martin Dunitz; 2000. p. 595–613.

[55] Peet RM, Henriksen JD, Anderson TP, et al. Thoracic-outlet syndrome: evaluation of a therapeutic exercise program. Mayo Clin Proc 1956;31:281–7.

[56] Lindgren K-A, Manninen H, Rytkönen H. Thoracic outlet syndrome—a functional disturbance of the thoracic upper aperture? Muscle Nerve 1995;18:526–30.

[57] Novak CB, Mackinnon SE. Thoracic outlet syndrome. Orthop Clin North Am 1996;27: 747–62.

[58] Crosby CA, Wehbé MA. Conservative treatment for thoracic outlet syndrome. Hand Clin 2004;20:43–9.

[59] Katz JN, Simmons BP. Carpal tunnel syndrome. N Engl J Med 2002;346:1807–12.

[60] Hui ACF, Wong S, Leung CH, et al. A randomized controlled trial of surgery vs steroid injection for carpal tunnel syndrome. Neurology 2005;64:2074–8.

[61] Armstrong T, Devor W, Borschel L, et al. Intracarpal steroid injection is safe and effective for short-term management of carpal tunnel syndrome. Muscle Nerve 2004;29:82–8.

[62] Spinner RJ, Amadio PC. Compression neuropathies of the upper extremities. In: Tubiana R, Amadio PC, editors. Medical problems of the instrumentalist musician. London: Martin Dunitz; 2000. p. 273–93.

[63] Winspur I. Nerve compression syndromes. In: Winspur I, Wynn Parry CB, editors. The musician's hand: a clinical guide. London: Martin Dunitz; 1998. p. 85–99.

[64] Roos DB. Thoracic outlet syndromes: symptoms, diagnosis, anatomy, and surgical treatment. Med Probl Perform Art 1986;1:90–3.

[65] Newmark J. Thoracic outlet syndromes: a non-surgeon's perspective for those caring for musicians. Work 1996;7:95–107.

[66] Roos DB. Transaxillary approach for first rib resection to relieve thoracic outlet syndrome. Ann Surg 1966;163:354–8.

[67] Wehbé MA, Leinberry CF. Current trends in treatment of thoracic outlet syndrome. Hand Clin 2004;20:119–21.

[68] Cherington M, Happer I, Machanic B, et al. Surgery for thoracic outlet syndrome may be hazardous to your health. Muscle Nerve 1986;9:632–4.

[69] Wilbourn AJ. Thoracic outlet syndrome surgery causing severe brachial plexopathy. Muscle Nerve 1988;11:66–74.

ELSEVIER
SAUNDERS

Phys Med Rehabil Clin N Am
17 (2006) 781–787

PHYSICAL MEDICINE
AND REHABILITATION
CLINICS OF
NORTH AMERICA

Focal Dystonia in Musicians

Theresa J. Lie-Nemeth, MD[a,b]

[a]Spaulding Rehabilitation Hospital, 125 Nashua Street, Boston, MA 02114, USA
[b]Harvard Medical School, 25 Shattuck Street, Boston, MA 02115, USA

Focal dystonia is an important neurological disorder that can impact the lives and careers of instrumental musicians. Also known as musicians' cramp, patients with this condition may complain of a loss of voluntary control in the hands or embouchure (oral musculature) when playing their instrument. Symptoms generally do not manifest during other activities. The disorder may progress over a period of time and then stabilize. Focal dystonia never resolves spontaneously. Rest usually does not alter the condition. If the disease progresses, involuntary movements such as extension of the fifth digit or flexion of digits two and three may occur whenever the musician plays the instrument. Later, symptoms may carry over into other activities such as typing or writing.

The diagnosis of focal dystonia is clinical, based on history and observation of the musician playing. Instrumental musicians typically present with complaints of incoordination in the fingers or hand. Pain is generally not a feature of the condition. Any pain that is present is likely secondary to movements made in attempt to compensate for the dystonia. In woodwind or brass musicians, symptoms such as stiffness, cramping, or fatigue may be seen in the muscles of the tongue, lips, or jaw. Frucht and colleagues described embouchure dystonia in 26 professional brass and woodwind players [1]. Patterns of abnormal movements included embouchure tremor, involuntary lip movements, and jaw closure. Unlike in focal hand dystonia, the embouchure dystonia occasionally spreads to other oral tasks.

Physical and neurological examinations are almost always normal. On observation of the musician playing, findings can be subtle and only may been seen in certain passages. In each affected musician, the hand behaves in a stereotypical fashion. Between individuals, however, the pattern of dystonia varies. Depending on the severity of impairment, the musician may be able to play certain repertoire fairly well, or he or she may be unable to play a relatively simple piece.

E-mail address: tlienemeth@partners.org

Treatment is primarily palliative and not curative. Options include retraining, splints, oral medications, and botulinum toxin injections. Schuele and Lederman surveyed string instrumentalists with focal dystonia to assess their long-term outcome [2]. Out of 21 violin and viola players, 18 responded. These musicians tried nerve decompression, physical therapy, retraining, anticholinergic medications, botulinum toxin, and splints to treat their dystonia. Only 38% were able to continue playing professionally. Jabusch and colleagues also studied the long-term outcome of 144 musicians with focal dystonia [3]. Their study found slightly better results, with 54% acknowledging improvement of symptoms. Thirty-three percent improved with trihexyphenidyl, 49% with botulinum toxin, 50% with pedagogical retraining, 56% with technical exercises, and 63% with ergonomic changes.

Epidemiology

Focal dystonia is not uncommon in performing arts medicine clinics. Brand-fonbrener established that approximately 5% of her patients had focal dystonia [4]. Lederman cited a similar percentage of 8%. Tubiana's clinic had 11% [5], and Newmark and Hochberg found 13% of their patients to have this condition [6].

Although focal dystonia can occur earlier or later in life, the peak incidence is in the fourth decade [4,7]. Seventy-five percent of those affected are men, regardless of the proportion of men playing a particular instrument. Professional musicians are affected primarily, presumably because it takes a high degree of exposure over time for this problem to occur. Although focal dystonia may occur in any type of instrumentalist, it is more common in musicians who play keyboards, strings, and woodwinds.

Pathophysiology

The pathophysiology for focal dystonia remains unknown, although some predisposing factors have been identified. Overuse may contribute to the development of the disorder [8]. Tension also could be a factor. Furthermore, biomechanical disadvantages in the hand, such as a small hand or small digit span, may lead to the development of dystonia. It is suggested that compensatory movements used may lead to the changes in cortical motor programs. Before the recent understanding of focal dystonia, clinicians attributed the patient symptoms to be psychological in nature. A psychological component still may contribute to the disorder. Jabusch and colleagues found a higher prevalence of anxiety and perfectionism in musicians with focal dystonia compared with musician controls [9].

Although the precise pathophysiology of the condition is unclear, it is known that the primary source of the problem is in the brain and not the peripheral nervous system. Transcranial magnetic source imaging has demonstrated a dedifferentiation in the finger representation in the somatosensory cortex [10]. That is, whereas in highly trained musicians the representation of each finger is well-delineated, in focal dystonia, the finger representation is less distinct.

Butterworth and colleagues confirmed abnormalities in the sensory cortex on functional MRI (f-MRI) [11]. They stimulated the index and fifth digits with vibration and analyzed the primary sensory cortex and other sensory areas. Compared with controls, dystonic subjects exhibited reduced separation between the finger representations. In addition, there was reversed ordering of representation in secondary sensory cortex and posterior parietal areas. Last, they noted underactivation in the secondary somatosensory cortex for both digits and in the posterior parietal area for digit five.

Pujol and colleagues also used f-MRI to study musicians, specifically guitarists, with focal dystonia. These dystonic guitarists were found to have larger activation of contralateral primary sensorimotor cortex and bilateral underactivation of premotor areas [12].

Garraux and colleagues studied patients with musicians' dystonia and those with writers' cramp, a focal hand dystonia akin to musicians' dystonia [13]. Using an MRI technique called voxel-based morphometry (VBM), patients who had dystonia had a bilateral increase in gray matter volume in the hand representation area of the primary somatosensory cortex, and to a lesser degree, the primary motor cortex, compared with controls. These findings support the idea that patients with focal dystonia have abnormalities of hand representation in the cerebral cortex.

Similarly, Blood and colleagues studied subjects with musicians' dystonia and writers' cramp [14]. f-MRI showed persisting elevations of basal ganglia activity after finger tapping. Their hypothesis is that in focal hand dystonia, inhibitory control of the basal ganglia may be problematic.

To tie together these aforementioned central nervous system findings, the following hypothesis has been suggested. In focal hand dystonia, there appears to be excessive motor cortical excitability with poor cortical sensory processing and dysfunctional mediation from the basal ganglia [15,16].

As for embouchure dystonia, Hirata and colleagues looked at the somatosensory homuncular representation using magnetoencephalography (MEG) [17]. They found that digit representations, especially the thumb, were shifted toward the lip representation region. On physical examination, the upper lips had decreased sensitivity compared with the lower lips. Perhaps this is because the upper lip is highly involved in vibration and production of rich sounds. In addition, when playing in a higher register, musicians often position the lower jaw slightly behind the upper jaw. As a result, the upper lips sustain higher pressure and compression. It is suggested that this decreased sensitivity may promote maladaptive cortical plasticity.

Evaluation

As previously stated, physical and neurological examinations are normal in patients who have focal dystonia. To best diagnose the condition, the physician needs to observe the musician while playing his or her instrument. Attention should be paid visually and aurally to the evenness of playing. In more severe cases, overt involuntary flexion and/or extension movements may be seen in the fingers. Symptoms may not be evident with simpler repertoire. The patient may notice more difficulties with certain types of passages, such as trills, arpeggios, or scales. The hand affected typically is the one that does the most work or is positioned in the most awkward way, such as the left hand in the violinist or flutist or the right hand in a pianist.

Several scales have been developed to rate the severity of dystonia. The Tubiana scale is as follows [18]:

0 Unable to play
1 Plays several notes but stops because of blockage or lack of facility
2 Plays short sequences without rapidity and with unsteady fingering
3 Plays easy pieces with restriction. Rapid sequences stir up motor problems.
4 Nearly normal playing but avoids technically difficult passages for fear of motor problems
5 Normal playing, returns to concert performances

The Arm Dystonia Disability Scale also is used frequently [19]:

0 Normal
1 Mild difficulty
2 Moderate difficulty
3 Marked difficulty

Candia and colleagues developed the Dystonia Evaluation Scale [20]:

0 Dystonia as bad as at its worst
1 Slightly improved
2 Moderately improved
3 Almost normal
4 Normal

Treatment

No treatment has been definitive for focal dystonia. Some musicians have found sensory tricks for themselves that help reduce symptoms. A sensory trick is a simple touch near the area of abnormal movement that decreases the dystonia [21]. Rest does not alter the course of the disease, although one group has tried treatment with limb immobilization [22]. Compensatory techniques can be attempted. Musicians may try to alter the repertoire, change fingerings, or potentially switch hands.

Various types of retraining also have been tried. Sakai described a slow-down exercise therapy that may be efficacious [23]. Zeuner and colleagues retrained subjects with writers' cramp [24]. These subjects underwent 4 weeks of retraining to decrease abnormal movements, resulting in mild subjective improvement. In this study, however, the motor cortex abnormalities seen in dystonia were not reversed on transcranial magnetic stimulation.

Sensory training also has been tried to treat writers with focal dystonia. Zeuner and Hallet had subjects learn Braille reading [25]. After training, there was improved spatial acuity and improvement in the dystonia.

Candia and colleagues have been successful with a variant of constraint-induced movement therapy [20]. More recently, they renamed their retraining technique "sensory motor retuning" (SMR) [26]. In their retraining process, one or more digits are immobilized with a splint. Subsequently, the focal dystonic finger participates in exercises with one or more of the nonsplinted digits. This retraining occurs for 8 consecutive days (1.5 to 2.5 h/d). Before retraining, somatosensory relationships in between the individual fingers differed between the affected and unaffected hands. After treatment, dystonic side became more similar to the less-affected side. Also after treatment, somatosensory finger representations were ordered more according to homuncular principles. Evaluation tools included a dexterity displacement device that provided spectral analysis of the evenness of playing, magnetoencephalography, and the Dystonia Evaluation Scale.

Medications such as anticholinergics (eg, trihexyphenidyl) have varied results and usually are limited by adverse effects. Botulinum toxin injections, though, can be effective in treating patients with focal dystonia. Schuele and colleagues reported that 69% of musicians found the injections beneficial, and 36% felt there was long-term benefit [27]. They used Dysport (Ipsen Limited, Berkshire, UK), botulinum toxin A, which is used widely in Europe. Dysport has a potency ratio of 1:3 compared with BOTOX (Allergan, Incorporated, Irvine, California). Average first dosage per muscle group was as follows:

Shoulder: 55 units (range 40 to 70)
Forearm flexors: 56 units (range 10 to 160)
Forearm extensors: 34.6 units (range 4 to 100)
Hand: 22.4 units (range 4 to 100)
Total dosage: 126.9 units (range 5 to 420)

Jabusch and colleagues listed the most commonly injected muscles for their musicians with focal dystonia [3]:

Flexor digitorum superficialis and flexor digitorum profundus (70% of patients treated with botulinum toxin)
Flexor carpi radialis (18%)
Flexor pollicis longus (10%)
Extensor digitorum (10%)
Extensor indicis (10%)
Interosseous palmaris (7%)

Limitations to botulinum toxin injections include weakness and antibody development.

Perhaps a multi-modal approach to treatment works best [5,8]. Physicians first should rule out nerve entrapment, and then consider trying oral medications. Additionally, they should encourage patients to learn relaxation and body awareness techniques, such as the Feldenkrais method or the Alexander technique. Technical re-education is important in addition to modifying playing technique. The physician may want to work with the musician's teacher to help the patient reduce tension and to maintain good ergonomics when playing. Splints that limit the dystonic movements could be tried also. Finally, if the musician is agreeable, botulinum toxin injections may be used judiciously. These treatments may be inadequate, however, so educating and counseling patients about the condition are extremely important.

Embouchure dystonia is even more challenging to treat than hand dystonia. With respect to medications, James and Cook have tried using bromocriptine [8]. From a behavioral standpoint, musicians could consider modifying their mouthpiece or performing retraining exercises for their embouchure.

In general, physicians should recommend healthy practices to their patients with focal dystonia, and to all of their musician patients. For example, musicians should avoid rapid increases in practice time or intensity. In addition, they should place a priority on reducing emotional stresses, tension, and anxiety. Healthy habits also include using warm-ups and cool-downs, taking breaks, maintaining general body conditioning, strength, and flexibility, and using good posture and ergonomics.

Summary

In conclusion, musicians' focal dystonia is a significant and potentially career-ending neurological condition of which physiatrists and other performing arts medicine clinicians should be aware. Pathology has been identified in the somatosensory cortex, and in the motor cortex and basal ganglia. Although advances have been made in the elucidating some of the pathologic changes in focal dystonia, better understanding is needed. Current treatments such as retraining, splinting, oral medications, and botulinum toxin injections are limited. Therefore, the ultimate goal for focal dystonia is to prevent this disabling disorder of instrumental musicians.

References

[1] Frucht SJ, Fahn S, Greene PE, et al. The nature history of embouchure dystonia. Mov Disord 2001;16(5):899–906.
[2] Schuele S, Lederman RJ. Long-term outcome of focal dystonia in string instrumentalists. Mov Disord 2004;19(1):43–8.
[3] Jabusch HC, Zschuke D, Schmidt A, et al. Focal dystonia in musicians: treatment strategies and long-term outcome in 144 patients. Mov Disord 2005;20(12):1623–6.

[4] Brandfonbrener AG, Robson C. Review of 113 musicians with focal dystonia seen between 1985 and 2002 at a clinic for performing artists. Adv Neurol 2004;94:255–6.

[5] Vargas-Rodriguez A, Kooh M, Amezcua-Guerra L, et al. Musician's Cramp: a case report and literature review. J Clin Rheumatol 2005;11(5):274–6.

[6] Newmark J, Hochberg FHH. Isolated painless manual incoordination in 57 musicians. J Neurol Neurosurg Psychiatry 1987;50:291–5.

[7] Brandfonbrener AG. Musicians with focal dystonia: a report of 58 cases seen during a ten-year period at a performing arts medicine clinic. Med Probl Perform Art 1995;10:121–7.

[8] Lederman RJ. Neurological problems of performing artists. In: Sataloff RT, Brandfonbrener AG, Lederman RJ, editors. Performing arts medicine. 2nd edition. San Diego (CA): Singular Publishing Group, Incorporated; 1998. p. 63–7.

[9] Jabusch HC, Muller SV, Altenmuller E. Anxiety in musicians with focal dystonia and those with chronic pain. Mov Disord 2004;19(10):1169–75.

[10] Elbert T, Candia V, Altenmuller E, et al. Alteration of digital representations in somatosensory cortex in focal hand dystonia. Neuroreport 1998;9:3571–5.

[11] Butterworth S, Francis S, Kelly E, et al. Abnormal cortical sensory activation in dystonia: an fMRI study. Mov Disord 2003;18(6):673–82.

[12] Pujol J, Roset-Llobet J, Rosinés-Cubells D, et al. Brain cortical activation during guitar-induced hand dystonia studied by functional MRI. Neuroimage 2000;12:257–67.

[13] Garraux G, Bauer A, Hanakawa T, et al. Changes in brain anatomy in focal hand dystonia. Ann Neurol 2004;55:736–9.

[14] Blood AJ, Flaherty AW, Choi JK, et al. Basal ganglia activity remains elevated after movement in focal hand dystonia. Ann Neurol 2004;55(5):744–8.

[15] Lederman RJ. Neuromuscular and musculoskeletal problems in instrumental musicians. Muscle Nerve 2003;27:549–61.

[16] Lim VK, Bradshaw JL, Nicholls ME, et al. Abnormal sensorimotor processing in pianists with focal dystonia. Adv Neurol 2004;94:267–73.

[17] Hirata Y, Schulz M, Altenmuller E, et al. Sensory mapping of lip representation in brass musicians with embouchure dystonia. Neuroreport 2004;15(5):815–8.

[18] Toledo SD, Nadler SF, Norris RN, et al. Sports and performing arts medicine. Issues relating to musicians. Arch Phys Med Rehabil 2004;85:S72–4.

[19] Jabusch HC, Vauth H, Altenmuller E. Quantification of focal dystonia in pianists using scale analysis. Mov Disord 2004;19(2):171–80.

[20] Candia V, Elbert T, Altenmueller E, et al. Constraint-induced movement therapy for focal hand dystonia in musicians. Lancet 1999;353(9146):42.

[21] Pullman SL, Hristova AH. Musician's dystonia. Neurology 2005;64:186–7.

[22] Priori A, Pesenti A, Cappellari A, et al. Limb immobilization for the treatment of focal occupational dystonia. Neurology 2001;57l:405–9.

[23] Sakai N. Slow-down exercise for the treatment of focal hand dystonia in pianists. Med Probl Perform Art 2006;21(1):25–8.

[24] Zeuner KE, Shill HA, Sohn YH, et al. Motor training as treatment in focal hand dystonia. Mov Disord 2005;20(3):335–41.

[25] Zeuner KE, Hallett M. Sensory training as treatment for focal hand dystonia: a 1-year follow-up. Mov Disord 2003;18(9):1044–7.

[26] Candia V, Wienbruch C, Elbert T, et al. Effective behavioral treatment of focal hand dystonia in musicians alters somatosensory cortical organization. Proc Natl Acad Sci U S A 2003; 100(13):7942–6.

[27] Schuele S, Jabusch HC, Lederman RJ, et al. Botulinum toxin injections in the treatment of musician's dystonia. Neurology 2005;64(2):341–3.

ELSEVIER
SAUNDERS

Phys Med Rehabil Clin N Am
17 (2006) 789–801

PHYSICAL MEDICINE
AND REHABILITATION
CLINICS OF
NORTH AMERICA

Common Musculoskeletal Problems in the Performing Artist

Pamela A. Hansen, MD*, Kristi Reed, MD

*Department of Physical Medicine and Rehabilitation, University of Utah,
768 E 4th Avenue, Salt Lake City, UT 84103, USA*

In this chapter we examine some of the musculoskeletal injuries unique to musicians and dancers. The cornerstone of treatment in this specialized patient population is the understanding that the injuries these artists sustain occur in the context of a distinctive lifestyle. This lifestyle demands extreme physical and emotional stressors that are far outside the normal range of standard occupations and even most competitive sports. Understanding and treating all aspects of the performer requires a highly specialized interdisciplinary team approach that appreciates all of the conditions that govern these patients' lives.

Musculoskeletal injury in the musician

Instrumental musicians are a special risk group for musculoskeletal injuries. A large percentage of them have problems related to playing their instruments using incorrect posture, nonergonomic technique, excessive force, overuse, and insufficient rest, which may in turn result in musculoskeletal injury. These injuries can be devastating, leading to pain, which can be artistically and professionally limiting, or even career ending, with deleterious effects on the musician's physical, emotional, and financial well-being. This chapter reviews risk factors for musculoskeletal injuries in musicians and the importance of understanding the whole person. Preventative strategies are introduced. Proper evaluation of musicians who have musculoskeletal complaints are addressed, and discussion of specific diagnosis and treatment options commonly seen in musicians are done using a problem-oriented approach.

Routine daily activities place demands on the body that may contribute to the development of a musculoskeletal injury. The large number of hours

* Corresponding author.
 E-mail address: Pamela.Hansen@hsc.utah.edu (P.A. Hansen).

musicians spend practicing, rehearsing, and performing predispose them to musculoskeletal injury; multiple studies have found that anywhere from 50% to 80% of musicians experience physical problems. Risk seems to be greatest in string players and keyboardists, likely due to the postural demands of these instruments. These instruments require constant rapid movement for prolonged periods at forces that may exceed the body's capabilities to repair without adequate recovery time. Signs and symptoms of injury may appear suddenly or they may develop gradually over weeks to months. Complaints often include pain, weakness, reduced range of motion, numbness, tingling, or loss of muscular control, which interferes with their playing. Pain often results in loss of speed, volume, or control making difficult pieces impossible to play. Symptoms may not always be as problematic during the causative, aggravating activity as they are after playing. Symptoms often progress to being painful during the activity and become more difficult to manage if treatment is not initiated early. As with any musculoskeletal injury model, prevention ideal through controlling the risk factors and recognizing and responding to early signs and symptoms. Unfortunately, it is common for dedicated performers to work through pain until they can no longer perform. At this late stage, the likelihood of full recovery diminishes, and the treatment process is more complex and disruptive to daily life.

Several risk factors may increase musculoskeletal injury in performing artists. Understanding these risk factors and finding ways to minimize them is the most effective way to prevent frustrating and potentially career-ending effects of musculoskeletal injury. For performers, the greatest risk of musculoskeletal injury occurs when changing a technique or using a new instrument and with prolonged playing with inadequate rest such as when preparing for a performance or perfecting a new, technically difficult piece. Risk factors can be broken down into environmental factors, physical demands, and personal characteristics. Environmental risk factors include cold temperature, confined space or layout of space, equipment, surfaces, and lighting. Physical demands include awkward postures, forceful exertion, repetition, long-duration activities with inadequate rest, and vibration. Personal characteristics include an individual's posture, strength, flexibility, endurance and comorbid health conditions. Poor nutritional status and psychological stress, which often accompany a challenging schedule, may also relate to injury risk or hinder healing.

Environmental risk factors may include playing in cool temperatures, inadequate lighting, poor instrument fit, inadequately maintained instruments, and improper surrounding environment. Cold temperatures reduce blood flow to the fingers and arms and can slow nerve conductions in the extremities. Inadequate lighting can influence a musician's ability to read music, resulting in altered posture and eyestrain. Selecting an environment that is properly heated and well lit is ideal, but not always possible. When the environment is not optimal, the musician should wear adequate clothing to keep the entire body warm to maintain adequate blood flow to the extremities. Gloves or fingerless gloves may help keep the hands warm. Warming the hands before playing is important. In a poorly lit environment, the use of portable lamps or battery-powered clip lights to illuminate music can be helpful. Changing instruments presents a situation in which there is a sudden change in physical demands and a resultant increase in the risk of musculoskeletal injury. Playing poorly maintained or poorly designed instruments can require greater effort or force than playing similar, well-maintained instruments. One common example of this would be wind instruments with leaky valves or pads and string instruments with bridges that are too high and require greater effort to play. Piano with excessive dead space at the tops of the keys will require more force to obtain volume. Choosing quality instruments and maintaining their proper working condition will assist in preventing musculoskeletal injury. Selecting an instrument that properly fits will assist the musician in adopting a reasonable playing posture without the need to adapt for excessive reaches or awkward hand and finger postures.

It is important to consider the surrounding environment, including chairs, music stands, and instrument stands to support the static weight of the instrument, which can have a profound influence on playing posture. Chairs should be at a height that allows the musician's feet to sit flat on the ground with the knees at a 90° angle. Chair cushions or footrests can accommodate alignment if a chair is an inappropriate height and not adjustable. Positioning of the music stand should place the top of the sheet music at or just below eye level. In addition to these general categories of risk factors, each musical instrument is associated with a unique set of injuries related to the physical and postural demands of playing that specific instrument. Evaluation and treatment as well as risk factor recognition and modification must therefore be musician and instrument specific. With such complex interplay, a multidisciplinary approach can serve this special patient population.

Overuse syndrome

Overuse syndrome or occupational overuse syndrome is a poorly defined and often incorrectly used term to define a constellation of symptoms of pain associated with activity and no specific diagnosis. The predominant feature of this syndrome is pain, and it is believed to be the most prevalent medical problem affecting musicians. Overuse syndrome is present in up to 50% of professional symphony orchestra musicians [1] and it accounts for 50% to 80% of consultations [2]. There may also be weakness or loss of fine motor control, but sensory symptoms are absent. Symptoms often develop after a change from the usual routine and may only be present just after or during performance. Any fluctuation in practice schedule involving a more difficult piece, prolonged playing times, inadequate rest periods, or touring can bring about an exacerbation. Factors known to contribute include physical disproportion between the instrument and the musician, poor posture, fatigue, excessive finger angulation, and biomechanical preconditions such as hypermobility or hypomobility of critical joints [3]. The common underlying pathology involves the tissues being stressed beyond their physiological limits; however, there is much debate as to the pathophysiology of this syndrome. Some investigators suggest that pathologic changes to peripheral tissues are involved, whereas others have proposed that the basis of symptoms is either fatigue or psychological pathology. There is certainly much debate as to the etiology and all of the contributing factors that make up this clinical picture. Currently, theories center on this entity as a protective mechanism occurring by some yet unknown physiologic process. When tissues are stressed, an unpleasant reaction is then set in motion that serves to limit the offending activity and therefore relieve the physiological stress [4]. In many cases, overuse syndrome is misdiagnosed bursitis, tendonitis, or other inflammatory conditions that can be shown to bring about histologic change. Investigations thus far have not shown overuse syndrome to bring about any of the histopathologic changes seen in inflammatory conditions.

Evaluation of the professional musician suspected of having overuse syndrome requires a detailed systematic observation of the musician and his interaction with his instrument. The patient should be undressed sufficiently for examination and should be assessed briefly for overall habitus, fitness, and posture. Any underlying disease should be noted. A full musculoskeletal examination should involve assessment of range of motion and strength of all joints of the upper limbs as well as the neck, shoulders, and spine. Any discomfort or reproduction of usual symptoms will aid in narrowing down the pain generator. Joints should also be assessed for hypermobility as well as hypomobility. Joint deformity as well as callous formation can be an indicator of poor technique. A full neurologic examination should include signs of muscle atrophy indicating possible neuropathy as well as sensation and reflexes. The patient should be examined playing their instrument in a manor that most closely resembles their usual playing style. With the musician performing, one may easily evaluate tension, pressure, and angulations of the painful area as well as all adjoining segments. Observations should also be made after a prolonged period of practice so that a comparison may be made as the musician fatigues. This can be accomplished easily with video taped sessions if observation is not practical in the office setting. A specifically trained physical or occupational therapist often can assist in biomechanical evaluation as well.

Treatment of overuse syndrome centers on relative rest. Because musicians have high anxiety associated with job uncertainty and extreme pressure to maintain standards of almost unattainable excellence, rest often is met with great resistance. In an attempt to have as little impact on career as possible, it is often helpful to involve coaches, conductors, music teachers, or managers. These professionals can advise realistic plans of rest periods and practice schedules that will help ensure patient compliance and overall treatment success. Investigators have reported more than 80% success rates of return to normal playing schedules [5] with relative rest and slow gradual rehabilitation. A good general guideline for treatment starts with ergonomic modification as well as instrument modification when possible. Straps can be used to help support the weight of a heavy instrument, keys on woodwind instruments may be altered for ease of fingering, and chair height and seating can be adjusted. The actual size of the instrument may be adjusted and can have a large impact on biomechanics. In some cases, a change may be beneficial. Blum and Ahlers [6] found a relationship between the size of the viola and shoulder problems. There is some variation in violas, and violists playing instruments greater than 40 cm in length are more likely to have shoulder pain. After ergonomic and postural adjustments, a detailed program of rest should be outlined and agreed on by musician, music teacher or conductor, and physician. Musical pieces that are less technically demanding should be used for practice sessions, and length of practice sessions and performances should be extended very gradually. Rest times vary by degree of injury, and the amount of rest needed can vary from days to months. When play resumes, optimizing proper warm up, relaxation training, hydration, proper diet, and physical conditioning can all aid in rehabilitation and injury avoidance. Physical therapy and occupational therapy with modalities as needed to get the patient through the acute phase may consist of heat, ice, transcutaneous electrical nerve stimulation, soft tissue mobilization, and ultrasound scan. Splinting may be used to decrease static or dynamic forces or to transfer force to adjacent structures; however, splinting actually may cause technical difficulties with performance and may actually cause injury to other unaffected joints. Nonsteroidal anti-inflammatory medications are often used; however, there is controversy concerning this practice as overuse syndrome is considered a noninflammatory condition. Local injections of steroids have been used with varied success.

Proper diagnosis and early management of overuse syndrome is not only essential in preventing loss of practice and performance time, but there is some evidence that there may be an association between overuse syndrome, complex regional pain syndrome (formerly, reflex sympathetic dystrophy), and focal dystonia. Lockwood and Lindsay [7] have reported an association between overuse syndrome, reflex sympathetic dystrophy (RSD), and focal dystonia. Their data support the early diagnosis of RSD because they believe that it may be the sensory analog of dystonia.

Focal motor dystonias

One of the more rare but perhaps most debilitating problems for the instrumentalist is focal motor dystonia. This is an insidious problem that develops over many years [8]. Focal motor dystonia is characterized best by painless spasm and involuntary movements in the affected limb. These movements are almost always aggravated by voluntary movement and may be apparent only during playing but in advanced cases may occur at rest [9]. In one series, Newmark and Hochberg looked at painless, uncoordinated movements in 57 musicians [10]. Their data suggest that the most commonly affected musicians were keyboard players (n = 35), followed by string players (n = 13), and woodwind players (n = 9). Their data also reflect that involuntary flexion of the fourth and fifth digit is the most common dystonia, with the right hand being more affected than the left. This condition has also been found to be more common in men with average age of onset at 38 years [11].

To date, the pathogenesis of focal motor dystonia is unknown, and there is no proven definitive treatment. Several theories as to etiology favor a central origin that is a function of excessive motor cortical excitability with poor cortical sensory processing and mediation from the basal ganglia [11]; still others suggest associations with multiple types of prior injury [7,10,12]. Some patients report that by producing sensory input such as touching the skin, or proprioreceptive input such as a small change in position, they can achieve temporary relief [9]. Permanent resolution of symptoms, however, is yet elusive, and possibly the most appropriate intervention is referral for psychological counseling because this condition often is career ending. Treatments tried without great success include steroids (both oral and local injections), prolonged rest, physical therapy, botulinum toxin, biofeedback, tricyclic antidepressant medications, immobilization, bromocryptine, and surgery. The importance of diagnosis cannot be understated, because this devastating condition may have an underlying biochemical, metabolic, genetic or anatomic etiologies that may benefit from more conventional treatments aimed at the specific condition. This has been found to be the case in up to 25% of the documented cases [13]. Appropriate diagnosis can spare the patient time, money, and often painful treatments that will most probably have limited success [14].

Osteoarthritis

Osteoarthritis, although a common condition in the general population, takes on special significance in the musical performer. Musicians depend on their bodies and specifically their hands for their livelihood. A typical professional musician has started his career at the age of 5 to 10 years, and many instrumentalists have full-time schedules well into their 70s [15]. Because osteoarthritis is the most common type of arthritis and increases with advancing age, it is commonly seen in the aging musician. The main complaint of the arthritic patient is pain, but joint stiffness and loss of range of motion are thought to be the most detrimental. The joints most commonly affected in the general population are the metacarpalphalangeal (MCP), distal interphalangeal (DIP), and carpometacarpal (CMC) joints of the hands, spine, hips, and knees. Data reporting as to whether musicians have a higher rate of degenerative arthritis in the hands and spine are sparse;

however, one might deduce that years of repetitive motion against static and dynamic stressors would elevate the incidence in this group.

Careful workup and diagnosis to rule out specific inflammatory conditions such as DeQuervain's tenosynovitis, overuse syndrome, and other rheumatologic conditions is warranted because treatment strategies differ. Signs and symptoms of osteoarthritis include dull aching pain that increases with playing and is relieved by rest, joint stiffness for less than 30 minutes, joint instability, and crepitus on range of motion. Patients may also report joint "gelling" which is perceived as a stiffness lasting short periods that dissipates after initial range of motion. Specific joint involvement includes spur formation at the DIP joints (Heberden's nodes) and at the PIP joints (Bouchard's nodes) as well as the first CMC joint. Radiographic findings include asymmetric narrowing of the joint space, subchondral bony sclerosis, osteophyte formation, and osseous cysts. It should be noted that no erosive changes should be seen. Marginal or central erosions are more consistent with rheumatoid arthritis.

Treatment is designed to protect the affected joint, alleviate painful symptoms, and restore range of motion. Once damaging playing techniques are recognized, they must be changed if long-term joint health is to be maintained. Prompt treatment of tendonitis and other inflammatory conditions prevents misuse of the joint and subsequent alterations in biomechanical forces. Splints may be used for relative rest and for joint instability; however, immobility that is prolonged causes demineralization of bone and muscle atrophy, whereas exercise has positive effects on collagen deposition tendon strength. There is a thin line between use and abuse in the osteoarthritic joint that the patient will ultimately have to balance. Musicians may be taught to play in joint midrange to aid in joint preservation. This position gives optimal balance between muscle stabilizers and active movers [16]. Patients should also be educated in proper warm-up techniques and may require external warming to alleviate stiffness before performances. Medications include, acetaminophen, nonsteroidal anti-inflammatory drugs, COX II inhibitors, and in rare cases narcotics. Data on glucosamine and chondroitin Sulfate are inconclusive at this point, and formulations in the United States are not regulated by the US Food and Drug Administration or standardized. In acute flair ups, intra-articular steroid injections may be used. In rare cases, surgical intervention including joint fusion and replacement may alleviate symptoms and still allow the technical level of performance desired.

Joint hypermobility

Joint hypermobility can be associated with connective tissue disorders such as Marfan's or Ehlers-Danlos syndrome or can be seen in isolation and identified as benign hypermobility. As in the general population, musicians often experience laxity at one or more joints and it may be present on examination of a painful or unstable joint. The question then is: is this pathologic? Is joint hypermobility an asset or a liability for instrumentalists? There is much debate on this subject. Studies such as the one performed by Larsson and colleagues [17] reported that based on observations of 660 musicians at music school, only 5% of the 96 musicians with hypermobility at the wrist reported pain and stiffness compared with the 18% of all other musicians. An opposing set of data from Brandfonbrener [18] based on studies of 393 musicians with hand and arm pain, found a prevalence of 19% joint laxity in her series suggesting laxity as a significant factor predisposing players to injury. Even with the contradictory evidence on hypermobility as a whole, it is clear that on an individual basis, excess joint laxity can be pathologic. Hypermobility can lead to instability of the loaded joint and, in turn, lead to the development of traumatic synovitis in instrumentalists. Hypermobility can also lead to digital nerve compression, and hyperextensibility of the wrist and elbow may contribute to neuropathy at these sights by exacerbating traction damage [19]. With joint laxity, muscle contraction then becomes the primary stabilization of the affected joint. Prolonged need for dynamic stabilization ultimately leads to fatigue, pain, and spasm when ligamentous structural support is lacking. This situation is seen commonly when woodwind players must bear the static load of the instrument on their thumb and in bass and cello players at the first MCP and CMC joints. Treatment is based on improving dynamic stability with increased muscle tone and endurance. This is best achieved with an occupational or physical therapist with specific knowledge in performing arts medicine. In cases in which there is gross instability or frank dislocation, dynamic splinting may be needed. In refractory cases, surgical reconstruction may be indicated. In the case of the thumb, the ulnar collateral ligament of the first MCP joint using a palmaris longus graft or plastic reconstruction of the CMC basal ligament can be used to create a stable functional joint [20].

Trauma

It goes without saying that accidents happen, and musicians are no exception. Trauma to the upper extremity comes in all forms and can account for a significant number of injuries to the instrumentalists. In one series, more than half of the injuries seen at a performance medicine clinic by an orthopedic surgeon were caused by trauma not associated with playing an instrument [19]. It is impossible to prevent all accidents and possible sources of trauma, but in a profession that demands precision and excellence beyond compare, patients must carefully weigh the risks and benefits of activities in which they participate.

Prevention

Ideally, we look to prevent injury and overuse. To completely prevent injury, however, we must know all of the causative factors. As stated previously, the interplay between individual musicians and their instruments combined with external stressors present an infinite number of variables to control and correct. More research is needed into all areas that affect this group of specialized patients. Awareness of obvious risk factors and comparative studies in specialized populations such as athletes, do help us generalize some basic principals. Prevention programs, however, no matter what area of medicine, are riddled with inherent problems. It is a difficult thing to motivate potential patients when they are feeling well. The constant demand for perfection and the high anxiety involved with job uncertainty, make this population especially vulnerable to the "play now, pay later" attitude. It is our job, together with music educators to help musicians and in particular young music students, to see that preventative strategies are in their best interests for a long and fulfilling musical career.

Musculoskeletal injuries in dancers

In great contrast to the long career of musicians are the short physically demanding and injury-prone years of the dancer. In this chapter we take a brief look at the most common musculoskeletal injuries encountered by the dancer and methods of evaluation, treatment, and prevention of injury.

In no other profession is the athlete more predisposed to injury than in ballet. Typically, professional ballerinas start at the age of 5 to 8 years and begin an immediate process of tremendous bodily strain. By 30, most have ended their career. If a female dancer is on track for a professional career, she may start dancing *sur les pointes,* or "on toe" at age 12. This unnatural position leads to tremendous forces being transmitted to the metatarsalphalangeal (MTP) and other joints. This and other unusual biomechanical stressors, combined with hypermobility, repetitive motion, delayed menarche, secondary amenorrhea, lack of job security, and the competitiveness of the dance company itself, makes the dancer an athlete like no other.

To live in the world of the professional ballerina, one must endure hours of physically demanding practice. The average weekly workload of the dancer is 45 hours, with only about one fifth of that time spent actually performing [21]. The competitiveness of the ballet company breeds an environment in which admission of injury can mean the end of a career. In this setting, injuries are reported late or not at all. When the affected part is then too painful for the dancer to continue, the injury often is at a much more advanced stage and more difficult to treat. For similar reasons, dancers may be inclined to return to full participation too soon and risk reinjury. Ironically, the dancer is the athlete most in need of full pain-free rehabilitation before full return to work. Elite dancers cannot perform at the artistic level needed without full recovery. Every angle and motion of the classical ballerina needs to be precise and perfect to convey the complete intention of the choreographer. Any deviation will be evident to the dancer, dance instructor, and audience but not necessarily the physician. For this reason, collaboration with instructors, therapists, and treating physicians is vital.

Common patterns of injury/lower extremity

Other chapters in this review detail lower extremity injuries in the dancer. In this chapter, our only intent is to highlight the unique needs of the dancer and to emphasize the importance of examining the patient in the context of her craft. More than 80% of ballet injuries involve the spine and lower extremities [22]. Looking at the lower extremities, en point dancers, as might be expected, have a high incidence of foot and ankle injuries. The exaggerated metatarsal arch produces bunions, hallux valgus, stiffness of the tarsal joints, and hammer toes. In the early phase of foot pain, modalities such as heat and ice in combination with rest, elevation, molded arch supports, and range of motion can alleviate pain. More often, however, injuries are more serious. Stress fractures are common and present as either focal or diffuse pain initially and then sharp pain in the final stages. The most common site for stress fractures in the dancer is the shafts of the 3 central metatarsals, and stress fractures of the anterior tibial cortex are common in performances that require many jumps. Because few stress fractures are evident on a plain radiograph, radioisotope bone scan done early will help in the diagnosis; however, even these have been known to be negative for the first few weeks [21].

Other lower limb injuries common to the dancer include ligamentous strains of the knee and ankle tendonopathies. Tendonitis of the flexor hallucis longus tendon at the posterior medial ankle can be especially disabling with the ankle in maximum dorsiflexion as in the plie position. Patellar dislocations are also common and are a consequence of the" turned out" position. This position puts the knee at a mechanical disadvantage for proper patellar tracking. Often this acute injury may be missed as the dancer reports to the physician with a painful swollen knee that obscures the patellar deformity. X-rays must be taken to ensure proper diagnosis and treatment [23]. Other common injuries include jumper's knee (patellar tendonitis), muscle strains, meniscal injuries, chondromalacia patellae, and other overuse injuries related to the excessive training demands [24].

Common spinal injuries

Flexibility is one of the hallmarks of the elite dancer, but it may be one of their greatest liabilities when it comes to spinal injury. The spine of the dancer is exposed to tremendous force at a great mechanical disadvantage. Similar to gymnasts, dancers experience high rates of spondylolysis and spondylolisthesis [25]. Spondylolysis is a vertebral defect at the pars interarticularis, which is at the junction of the pedicle, transverse process, lamina, and 2 articular processes. Spondylolisthesis, forward or backward slippage of one vertebral body on the other, may occur owing to pars defect or fractures. Hyperextension, in combination with jumping and heavy lifts, expose the dancer to increased risk for these injuries. The pars interarticularis is more vulnerable to trauma in the hyperlordotic and hyperextended position, and in women, the pars interarticularis is especially at risk. Female dancers begin their training before the epiphyseal union of this structure, and this makes spondylolysis more likely [21]. Hypermobility combined with repetitive stress causes microfractures that ultimately lead to stress fractures. This action puts all of the posterior spinal elements at risk. Stress fractures of the facet joints are not uncommon and can mimic spondylolysis [26].

Symptoms of spondylolysis include low back pain during strenuous practice or performance. Pain is localized lateral to midline and is reproduced with rotation and hyperextension of the lumbar spine. There may be tenderness of the paravertebral musculature and a positive spinal instability test. Further workup should include radiographic studies that include AP, lateral, and oblique views of the lumbar spine. If spinal films are negative, and clinical suspicion exists, technetium polyphosphate scan should be done and can elucidate stress fractures long before standard radiographs [25]. Treatment of spondylolysis includes relative rest, including a neutral spine-strengthening program such as Pilates, epidural steroid injections, and aquatic therapy. The dancer should continue with flexibility exercises and activity that does not aggravate symptoms. If there is pain with activities of daily living, bracing may be necessary. Spondylolisthesis or slippage of the actual vertebral body is measured in terms of percentage displacement seen on radiograph (Box 1).

Symptoms are similar to those for spondylolysis; however, radicular symptoms may be apparent if vertebral displacement is marked. Treatment for grades 1, 2, and asymptomatic grade 3 spondylolisthesis is conservative and similar to treatment for spondylolysis. Close clinical and radiographic monitoring is necessary for signs of increasing degree of slippage. For symptomatic grade 3 and above, surgical stabilization is warranted.

Other pain generators in the spine include sacroiliac, discogenic, and myofascial back pain. Evaluation of these is similar to those in the general population; however, as stated previously, they are more likely to present in a more advanced state. Rehabilitation may depend more on looking for relative strength and flexibility deficits rather than absolute deficiencies.

Box 1. Grading spondylolisthesis

Grade 0: 0% slip
Grade 1: <25% slip
Grade 2: 25–50% slip
Grade 3: 50–75% slip
Grade 4: 75–100% slip

Dancers are known for their strong core and extreme flexibility, which are usually the first targets for physical therapy aimed at generalized low back pain. Once again, therapists and physicians who can examine the dancer in context and seek out and correct relative imbalance are more likely to be successful in long-term management.

Prevention: physical environmental hazards

As is the case in musicians, often the physical environment of the dancer is outside her control. Great gains have been made in studio floor design and climate control, but often performances are outside in extreme cold and heat. It is essential for dancers to properly warm up in conditions of cold temperatures and stay well hydrated in environments of heat and humidity. Dance floors in amphitheaters and historical theaters often are of poor quality with respect to shock absorption. The ideal dance surface is one that absorbs some energy but is not too springy. Studies done on various highly resilient surfaces have reported a decrease in musculoskeletal injuries upwards of 80% [27].

Resting when able to avoid overuse and treating injuries early are still ideas that are difficult to convey to young dancers. These, unfortunately, are only a few of the methods that are under the direct control of the dancer. Careful attention to preventative strategies and early treatment will certainly aid in a pain-free and successful career.

Summary

In this chapter we touched on a wide variety of unique musculoskeletal conditions in the musician and dancer. We outlined generalized methods of evaluation that stress the importance of the interdisciplinary approach in this highly specialized patient population and stressed the importance of specific involvement of the music or dance instructor in evaluation and management. We sought to emphasize the need to refer to specialized care early when in doubt of diagnosis or when usual first-line treatments fail. We gave examples of specific injury patterns common in these subgroups and suggestions for early management. Finally, we described some general principals for prevention of musculoskeletal injury in this group. A physician treating the performing artist must always keep in mind that in this unique patient population, their occupation is not only a means of earning a living, it is their passion. Artists make great sacrifice both physically and mentally to bring the world such immeasurable beauty. It is our responsibility to care for them in the most comprehensive and compassionate manner possible while informing them as honestly as possible about their treatment options.

References

[1] Fry HJH. Incidence of overuse syndrome in the symphony orchestra. Med Probl Perform Art 1986;1:51–5.

[2] Dawson HJ. Hand and upper extremity problems in musicians; epidemiology and diagnosis. Med Probl Perform Art 1988;3:19–22.

[3] Wilson F, Wagner C, Hömberg V, et al. Interaction of biomechanical and training factors in musicians with occupational cramp/focal dystonia. Neurology 1991;4(suppl 1):291–2.

[4] White JW, Hayes MG, Jamieson CG. A search for the pathophysiology of the nonspecific "occupational overuse syndrome" in musicians. Hand Clin 2003;19(2):331–41.

[5] Knishkowy B, Lederman RJ. Instrumental musicians with upper extremity disorders: a follow up study. Med Probl Perform Art 1986;1:85–9.

[6] Blum J, Ahlers J. Ergonomic considerations in violists' left shoulder pain. Med Probl Perform Art 1994;9:25–9.

[7] Lockwood AH, Lindsay ML. Reflex sympathetic dystrophy after overuse: the possible relationship to focal dystonia. Med Probl Perform Art 1989;4:114–7.

[8] Lockwood AH. Medical problems of musicians. N Engl J Med 1989;320:221–7.

[9] Fahn S. Dystonia: phenomenology, classification, etiology, genetics, and pathology. Med Probl Perform Art 1991;6:110–5.

[10] Newmark J, Hochberg FH. Isolated painless manual incoordination in 57 musicians. J Neurol Neurosurg Psychiatry 1987;50:291–5.

[11] Lederman RJ. Neuromuscular and musculoskeletal problems in instrumental musicians. Muscle Nerve 2003;27:549–61.

[12] Lederman RJ. Occupational cramp in instrumental musicians. Med Probl Perform Art 1988; 3:45–51.

[13] Marsden CD. Investigation and treatment of dystonia. Med Probl Perform Art 1991;6: 116–21.

[14] Toledo SD, Nadler SF, Norris RN, et al. Sports and performing arts medicine.5. Issues relating to musicians. Arch Phys Med Rehabil 2004;85(3, suppl 1):S72–4.

[15] Hoppmann RA, Ekman E. Arthritis in the aging musician. Med Probl Perform Art 1999;14: 80–4.

[16] Ostwald PF, Baron BC, Byl NM, et al. Performing arts medicine. West J Med 1994;160(1): 48–52.

[17] Larsson LG, Baum J, Mudholkar GS, et al. Benefits and disadvantages of hypermobility among musicians. N Engl J Med 1993;329:1079–82.

[18] Brandfonbrener AG. Joint laxity in instrumental musicians. Med Probl Perform Art 1990;5: 117–9.

[19] Dawson WJ. Experience with hand and upper extremity problems in 1,000 instrumentalists. Med Probl Perform Art 1995;10:128–33.

[20] Nolan WB. Surgical management of acquired hand problems. In: Bejjani FJ, editor. Current research in arts medicine. Chicago: A Capella Books; 1993. p. 319–22.

[21] Garrick JG, Lewis SL. Career hazards for the dancer. Occup Med 2001;16(4):609–18.

[22] Garrick JG, Requa RK. An analysis of epidemiology and financial outcome. Am J Sports Med 1993;21(4):586–90.

[23] Quirk R. Knee injuries in classical dancers. Med Probl Perform Art 1988;3:52–9.

[24] Kelly KR. Injury in ballet: a review of relevant topics for the physical therapist. J Orthop Sports Phys Ther 1994;19(2):121–9.

[25] Keene JS, Drummond DS. Mechanical back pain in the athlete. Compr Ther 1985;11(1): 7–14.

[26] McCormack RG, Athwal G. Isolated fracture of the vertebral articular facet in a gymnast: a spondylolysis mimic. Am J Sports Med 1999;27(1):104–6.

[27] Washington EL. Musculoskeletal injuries in theatrical dancers: site, frequency and severity. Am J Sports Med 1978;6(2):75–97.

ELSEVIER
SAUNDERS

Phys Med Rehabil Clin N Am
17 (2006) 803–811

PHYSICAL MEDICINE
AND REHABILITATION
CLINICS OF
NORTH AMERICA

Dance Medicine: Current Concepts

Clay Miller, MD, MFA

Performing Arts Medicine, Boston University Medical School,
Sports Medicine North, 1 Orthopedics Drive, Peabody, MA 01960, USA

Dance medicine has grown exponentially over the past 10 to 15 years and continues to grow every year as more former professional dancers and students of dance enter into the field of medicine. Dance medicine is part of the field of performing arts medicine, which specializes in evaluating and treating performing artists such as musicians, dancers, actors/actresses, and vocalists. There are many different physician specialties involved with this field, including physiatrists, neurologists, orthopedists, rheumatologists, otolaryngologists, and psychiatrists along with physicians of internal medicine, family medicine, and occupational medicine. There are also many different allied health clinic professionals involved with treating these artists, including physical and occupational therapists, chiropractors, acupuncturists, nutritionists, and practitioners of Pilates, Feldenkrais and Alexander methods. In addition, there are many different forms of dance, including classical ballet, modern, jazz, tap, flamenco, folk dance, and ballroom dancing. Classical ballet originated in Italy during the Renaissance period and continued to flourish when taken to France by Catherine de Medici. This form of dance was an outgrowth of three popular pastimes of the nobility, including fencing, dancing and horsemanship. Dancing on pointe (on the toes) began in the early 1800s. This technique has separated classical ballet from all other dance forms both technically and medically. This article reviews the literature on dance medicine for various health-related medical issues, for the types of injuries commonly found, for the common surgical and rehabilitation interventions, and for injury prevention used in this unique group of patients.

The art of dance, particularly ballet, is one of the most physically demanding activities on the musculoskeletal system. Most literature and medical treatments focus on professional classical ballet and professional modern dance probably because of the high injury rate. Sixty-seven percent

---

E-mail address: cmiller@sportsmednorth.com

1047-9651/06/$ - see front matter © 2006 Elsevier Inc. All rights reserved.
doi:10.1016/j.pmr.2006.06.005

to 95% of the company dancers per year average approximately 1.7 to 6.7 injuries per dancer per contract year [1–4]. Overuse injuries remain the most common type of reported injury, with the highest incidence in the foot and ankles followed by the hip, lumbar/thoracic/cervical spine, and then knee/leg [1–6]. This is because of the sheer nature of their physical activity. Dance classes can last up to 1.5 hours followed by rehearsals that can last up to 5 hours. The dancer's body can be exposed to a highly physical demanding activity for greater than 6 hours per day. Many dancers also may have only 1 day of rest per week. In addition, the workload increases during beginning of a performance season such as the Nutcracker, which is performed the most each year (as many as 30 performances), or when returning to work after a relative time off from dance [3]. Age and gender do not appear to increase the risk for injury, which appears more related to high-level physical demand on the individual [7]. Thus, injury prevention has focused on educating the performer, teachers, and staff to modify activity levels to allow for adequate rest and recovery time for the dancer's body.

Most of the literature on dance injuries comes from studies on professional companies. There are some published studies on the students of dance from various performing arts schools showing differing injury rates per school year, from 47.3% by the Robson study [8], 49% by the Hamilton study [9], and 19.5% by the Miller study [10]. These studies found that nonmusculoskeletal health-related problems of stress and anxiety were reported as having a significant negative effect on performance. These psychosocial stressors were shown to have an adverse effect on the dancer physically and to contribute to a higher injury rate. Dancers who undergo psychosocial stress-related interventions have been shown to have less physical injuries and increased recovery from injuries [11,12]. This is an emerging field of medicine focusing on treating the psyche. Further research is needed to advance this area of intervention for injury prevention and treatment of injuries in dancers.

Another important health-related issue includes the female athlete triad, which needs to be considered in the young dancer because of the higher prevalence of late menses in this group. Today's classical ballet dancer is at least 20 lbs lighter than her counterpart of 40 plus years ago. Thinness is considered desirable aesthetically for the female dancer. Such focus easily leads to eating disorders, and medical practitioners often overlook the nutritional needs of their patients. Several Studies show that at least 6.5% of the female dancers suffer from eating disorders such as anorexia and bulimia, and up to 22% suffer from other nonspecified eating disorders [13,14]. This is followed by amenorrhea and osteoporosis that collectively are known as the female athlete triad. The incidence is around 15% to 65% in athletes [15–17]. A similar rate has been found in female dancers [18]. The long-term effects of developing osteoporosis in younger women are serious, because they will deal with the complications of osteoporosis the rest of their lives. In addition, there is evidence that the risk of developing scoliosis occurs with the female athlete triad [19]. The female dancer has many of the common characteristics of the female athlete triad, which includes perfectionist personality, highly competitive, self-critical, lean physique, stress fractures without a change in activity, and recurrent stress fractures and young age. Early detection and intervention of these emerging characteristics is extremely important for injury prevention and health maintenance of the female dancer.

Many other factors contribute to dance injuries, including foot morphology, the dancer's physique, dance floor surfaces, footwear, training and technique errors, and poor nutrition [20–24]. Because these art-specific factors are not taught in medical schools or included in a typical rotation of a residency training program, the health care provider who wants to treat dancers really needs to have a good foundation of knowledge in this art form. This includes understanding ballet and dance technique, the language of dance, the psychosocial stress of this field, the specific health-related issues of this field, and the working situations of this field. Former dancers who have gone into medicine or the health care field have helped to bring their knowledge of the arts to the field of medicine. Physiatry, sports medicine, and orthopedics help provide the musculoskeletal medicine basis for treatment of dancers. The physician who does not have a dance background has to learn these other aspects of dance medicine through continuing education programs offered at arts medicine conferences, by studying the arts medicine literature, by working with dance teachers and dance educators, and by doing clerkships at the various arts medicine clinics.

Dance is a mix of art and athleticism, and dancers possess unique physical and anatomical qualities. They require specific flexibility and strength qualities of the body that are unique to the art form. Dancers are hyperflexible but not necessarily hypermobile [1,25,26]. Their flexibility is important to perform the classical ballet technique. For example, in order for female dancers to do pointe work (dancing on their toes with a supportive shoe), they require 90° of plantar flexion and 45° of great toe dorsiflexion [2,21,27]. Dancers require hip external rotation greater than 45° for adequate turnout, as 60% of turnout occurs at the hips, and 40% occurs from the knees and feet [2,28]. Dancers who are hypermobile are more injury prone, as the ligamentous laxity places increased demand on the stabilizing and supporting structures of the body's joints.

Increased flexibility comes from years of stretching the hamstrings and the spine both in extension and flexion. They do not necessary have increased hip range of motion as compared with nondancers, but they do have increased flexibility in the knees and feet [2,21,25–28]. All of these characteristics need careful attention during the evaluation and treatment of dancers.

Most of the research has documented the foot and ankle complex as the most commonly injured site in the dancer. Several foot pathologies can be seen mostly in female ballet dancers because of their pointe work. These pathologies include hallux valgus, claw toes, hammer toes, bone spurs, stress fractures (metatarsals most common), corns, and calluses. The metatarsal stress fractures usually involve the second metatarsal and occasionally Lisfranc's joint [29,30]. This joint is formed by the medial and lateral cuneiforms that surround the base of the second metatarsal, locking it into place, which increases stress to this bone. Traumatic fractures also occur, including the Jone's fracture and short oblique (dancer's) fracture [31]. The best foot morphology for the dancer is the peasant foot, where the first three toes are equal length along with a flat forefoot and sturdy arch. The Grecian (Morton) foot with the short first ray increases the dancer's risk of second metatarsal stress fractures. Other foot and ankle problems encountered include sprains, Achilles tendonitis, flexor hallucis tendonitis, plantar fasciitis, anterior and posterior impingement syndromes of the talus, and Os trigonum [32,33].

The most common knee injuries tend to be patellofemoral syndrome or anterior knee pain. Jumper's knee, shin splints, and subluxing patella follow in frequency. Traumatic injuries such as anterior cruciate ligament, medial collateral ligament, and meniscal and lateral collateral ligament tears occur, but less frequently. In the hip, dancers often complain of pain and clicking while performing develop (lifting the leg to above 90° of flexion or abduction). This can be caused by a mechanical issue of the iliofemoral ligament (Bigelow) or tendons of the iliopsoas and rectus femoris with the lesser trochanter. In addition, iliopsoas tendonitis/apophysitis or less commonly rectus femorus tendonitis/apophysitis can be potential causes for this condition. Thigh or groin strains commonly occur also. Less common are avulsion fractures of the sartorius and rectus femorus origins.

Low back pain in the dancer usually derives from muscular strains, but, because of the extreme hyperlordosis used to extend the spine, dancers have an increased rate of stress fractures of the posterior elements, particularly pars defects or spondylolysis. Spondylolisthesis and disc herniations are rare occurrences.

Dancers are extremely well-conditioned athletes. They have excellent muscle definition because of their low body fat (women less than 15% of ideal body weight) and acquired strength [2]. Their art form demands anaerobic metabolism and aerobic capacity. The strength developed to perform ballet is highly exercise-specific. There is some controversy in the literature as to whether dancers are stronger than other athletes. One study of knee strength showed dancers falling in between athletes and controls, while another study showed no significant difference in knee and foot strength from controls [27]. Methods for measuring strength, however, are not standardized, so drawing significant conclusions is difficult. One thing is certain; a female basketball player does not have the foot strength to do pointe work, and the female ballet dancer does not have the aerobic endurance to play a basketball game. This emphasizes the need to provide exercise-specific rehabilitation or strength conditioning to achieve the desired physical ability.

Because of the multiple facets of dance medicine, treating dancers has become multi-disciplinary. The arts medicine physician works with the dancer, parents, teachers, dance educators, surgeons, physical therapists, chiropractors, massage therapists, acupuncturists, and Pilates, Alexander, and Feldenkrais [34] therapists. Pilates has become the most popular exercise form used by dancers. Joseph H. Pilates, a boxer and weight lifter, developed a series of exercises to strengthen the core or body's center of the abdomen and spine. There are a series of floor exercises and machines developed to aid in resistive strength and flexibility training. The reformer, trap table, and chair can be used to rehabilitate dancers after an injury. These machines allow the dancer to perform exercises specific to their ballet technique, both non-weight-bearing and advancing to weight-bearing as tolerated. The addition of a series of springs allows for resistive strength training. The healthy dancer also can use the entire Pilates exercise program as cross-training during their active season and for maintenance of their physical condition on their off seasons. Although there is little published medical literature on Pilates, there is evidence of reduced pressures on the legs and feet with dance-specific exercises [35,36]. Because funding is limited in the arts for medical research, additional studies focusing on Pilates likely will remain limited. Most arts medicine specialists, physical therapist clinics, and ballet companies, however, already generally have accepted Pilates as a standard of care and have incorporated this exercise therapy form into their practices.

Other forms of rehabilitation also exist for dancers, including the Feldenkrais method and Alexander technique. Both forms use imagery and sensory feedback from the therapist and help with muscle relaxation and neuromuscular re-education. Both forms help the dancer to unlearn improper use of muscle functions and rehabilitate the body to use muscles correctly in the proper alignment and technique. More in-depth discussion on these modalities is available elsewhere [21,34].

In general, treatment considerations for most dance injuries typically focus on exhausting all conservative methods with rest or relative rest, ice, heat, nonsteroidal anti-inflammatory drugs, and other analgesic medications. In addition, use of PT modalities such as ultrasound, electrical stimulation therapies, iontophoresis, prolonged stretching, and therapeutic exercises is common. Therapeutic exercises should include dance technique-specific exercises. It also may be necessary to work with dance teachers to help modify ballet technique and work habits. The most common ballet technique faults include rolling in of the feet (foot eversion), forcing the turnout at the knees and feet, lifting heels off the floor in plie or when jumping, gripping the floor with the toes, hyperextending the back (sway back), tucking under of the pelvis, and not keeping the knee over the second toe in plie [21,27].

Although the most common types of dance injuries include overuse syndromes, traumatic injuries can occur. Dancers usually sustain sprains, strains, tendonitis, bursitis, and stress fractures. Other less common injuries include internal derangement of the knee injuries such as anterior cruciate ligament (ACL) tears and meniscal tears, along with tendon ruptures and disc herniations. The incidence of these types of injuries is reported as very low, with an average of five per year over 3 years [37]. Surgical options are typically the last resort for most dance injuries. The most common are those for traumatic type of injuries such as ACL tears, meniscal tears, tendon repairs (Achilles), tendon debridements (flexor hallucis longus) [33,38], removal of bone spurs, and occasional spine surgery for a disc herniation. Again, it is important to find surgeons who are familiar with the dancer's body and dance technique needs. Surgery and postoperative rehabilitation need to maintain or restore the dancer's unique range of motion and strength for full functional return to his or her particular art form. Pilates and pool therapy are useful tools in helping restore function of the dancer after surgery.

After reviewing all these injury characteristics of the dancer and their dance-specific interventions, one of the main goals of dance medicine over the past several years has been injury prevention. This has become a main focus for the future also. Injury prevention is important to pursue at an early age with the dancer, even at the grade school level, and it should continue throughout the dancer's career. Even with today's knowledge of the published literature on dance medicine, many ballet schools and touring ballet companies do not have optimal conditions that would help to prevent injuries. They do not have correct floor surfaces or teach the correct dance technique. Additionally, they have inadequate warm-up space. Even large touring music theater productions such as the Phantom of the Opera, which uses dancers with ballet technique, face the same suboptimal conditions to help protect the dancer from injury. Many of the theaters on these tours are not designed for the dancers' physical needs. Because of these issues, modification of activities and environment is important for the dancer to learn. The following tips can help:

- Proper warm-up/cool-down before dancing. Dancers can use heat to warm up muscles/tendons and gently stretch calves, hamstrings, quadriceps, hips, and low back. Do for 5 to 10 minutes. Prolonged stretches greater than 30 seconds after class for all muscles. Ice sore areas 20 minutes or 5 minutes of ice massage.
- Muscle soreness that goes away after 5 to 10 minutes is okay. Pain lasting longer may lead to injury. Sharp pain or persistent pain may indicate possible injury requiring rest and medical attention.
- Avoid hard dance surfaces or obtain proper sprung flooring.
- Proper fitting footwear and possible inserts/shoe modifications
- Proper nutrition (includes 1200 mg calcium with 800 U vitamin D for females)
- Proper ballet technique. Avoid rolling in off feet; do not force turn-out. Keep heels on the floor in plie; do not grip floor with toes. Do not hyperextend the back (sway back); do not tuck under pelvis. Keep the knee over the second toe.
- Avoid recreational activities that may add stress to the body.
- Counseling for stress management and eating disorders

Additional data on the student dancer level and professional dancer level would help tailor these preventive measures. Few published studies scientifically document if these preventative dance medicine measures help reduce dance injuries. It has been shown that injuries can be reduced (and medical insurance premiums) for a professional ballet company with a self-insured and company-based medical clinic on site [3]. The feasibility of replicating this type of system with other professional dance companies and ballet schools remains to be determined. More research is needed on the outcomes of preventative medicine for dancers. Comparing these outcomes with previous published research will help dance medicine specialists gain better insights on what preventative measures actually work for the entire field of dance.

Future considerations

Because of the numerous groups of professionals involved with the care of the performing artists, various arts medicine organizations have been developed around the world for the sharing of research, education, health maintenance/prevention, and developing common practice guidelines. Some of these organizations include the Performing Arts Medicine Association, (PAMA, United States), the International Association for Dance Medicine & Science (IADMS, United States), the British Arts Medicine Association (BAMA), the German Performing Arts Medicine Group (GPAMG), the Italian Performing Arts Medicine Group (IPAMG), and the National Dance Association (United States). These organizations combine memberships from all professionals in the field of arts medicine and have yearly conferences. Most have Web sites accessible by common links found on the Web site of www.artsmed.org. The dance medicine field needs to do a better job of standardizing research approaches to better quantify therapeutic techniques and injury prevention outcomes. This information is vital to the future for providing the highest quality of care for this specialized field of medicine. The Internet is a useful research tool, and it is being developed to provide communication around the world with arts medicine specialists. Hard-to-find arts medicine literature also can be found through these sites. Further development of preventative medicine techniques and education/health promotion is needed to pursue further areas, including nutrition, substance abuse, HIV, dance floors, protective footwear, activity modifications, and training errors. The dancers and their educators need to play active roles by following injury prevention and health promotion guidelines, along with helping to direct health care providers to their specific needs.

References

[1] Garrick JG, Requa RK. Ballet injuries. An analysis of epidemiology and financial outcomes. Am J Sports Med 1993;21(4):586–90.

[2] Hamilton WG, Hamilton LH, Marshall P, et al. A profile of the musculoskeletal character-istics of elite professional ballet dancers. Am J Sports Med 1992;20(3):267–73.

[3] Solomon R, Solomon J, Micheli LJ, et al. The cost of injuries in a professional ballet com-pany: A five year study. Med Probl Perform Art 1999;14:164–9.

[4] Bronner S, Ojofeitimi S, Rose D. Injuries in a modern dance company: effect of compre-hensive management on injury incidence and time loss. Am J Sports Med 2003;31(3): 365–9.

[5] Quirk R. Ballet injuries: the Australian experience. Clin Sports Med 1983;2(3):584.

[6] Washington EL. Musculoskeletal injuries in theatrical dancers: Site, frequency and severity. Am J Sports Med 1978;6(2):80–3.

[7] Garrick JG, Requa RK. The relationship between age and sex and ballet injuries. Med Probl Perform Art 1999;12(3):79–82.

[8] Robson BE, Gitev M. Health and health-related problems of art students. Med Probl Per-form Art 1993;8(4):136–40.

[9] Hamilton LH. Dancers' health survey, part II. From injury to peak performance. Dance Magazine 1997;60–5.

[10] Miller CD, Moa G. A retrospective epidemiological study of injuries sustained at a perform-ing arts school and the treatment outcomes. Med Probl Perform Art 1998;13(3):120–4.

[11] Young-Eun Noh, Morris T. Designing research-based interventions for the prevention of in-jury in dance. Med Probl Perform Art 2004;19(2):82–9.

[12] Mainwaring L, Kerr G, Krasnow D. Psychological correlates of dance injuries. Med Probl Perform Art 1993;8(1):3–6.

[13] Schnitt JM, Schnitt D. Eating disorders in dancers. Med Probl Perform Art 1986;1(2): 39–44.

[14] Ravaldi C, Vannacci A, Zucchi T, et al. Eating disorders and body image disturbances among ballet dancers, gymnasium users and body builders. Psychopathology 2003;36(5): 247–54.

[15] Drummer GM. Pathogenic weight control behaviors of young competitive swimmers. Phys Sportsmed 1987;115(5):75–86.

[16] Garner DM, Rosen LW, Barry D. Eating disorders among athletes. Research and recom-mendations. Child Adolesc Psychiatr Clin N Am 1998;7(4):839–57.

[17] Rosen LW. Pathogenic weight control behavior in female athletes. Phys Sportsmed 1986; 14(1):79–86.

[18] Koutedakis Y, Jamurtas A. The dancer as a performing athlete: physiological consider-ations. Sports Med 2004;34(10):651–61.

[19] Warren MP, Brooks-Gunn J, Hamilton LH, et al. Scoliosis and fractures in young dancers. Relation to delayed menarche and secondary amenorrhea. N Engl J Med 1986;314(21): 1348–53.

[20] Miller CD, Paulos LE, Parker RD, et al. The ballet technique shoe: A preliminary study of eleven differently modified ballet technique shoes using force and pressure plates. Foot Ankle 1990;11(2):97–100.

[21] Miller CD, Bengtson K. Performing arts medicine, physical medicine and rehabilitation: the complete approach. Blackwell Science; 1999.

[22] Hamilton LH, Hamilton WG. Occupational stress in classical ballet dancers: The impact in different cultures. Med Probl Perform Art 1994;9(2):35–8.

[23] Solomon RL, Trepman E, Micheli LJ. Foot morphology and injury patterns in ballet and modern dancers. Kinesiology and Medicine for Dance 1990;12(1):20–40.

[24] Werter R. Dance floors: a causative factor in dance injuries. J Am Podiatr Med Assoc 1985; 75(7):355–8.

[25] Grahame R, Jenkins JM. Joint hypermobility—asset or liability? A study of joint mobility in ballet dancers. Ann Rheum Dis 1972;31(109):109–11.

[26] Klemp P, Stevens JE, Isaacs S. A hypermobility study in ballet dancers. J Rheumatol 1984; 11(5):692–6.

[27] Bejjani FJ. Performing artist's occupational disorders. In: Delisa JA, editor. Rehabilitation medicine. Principles and practice. 2nd edition. Philadelphia: J.B. Lippincott Company; 1993. p. 1182–90.

[28] Garrick JG, Requa RK. Turnout and training in ballet. Med Probl Perform Art 1994;9(2): 43–9.

[29] Hamilton WG. Foot and ankle injuries in dancers. Clin Sports Med 1988;7(1):143–73.

[30] Kravitz SR, Huber S, Ruziskey JA, et al. Biomechanical analysis of maximal pedal stress during ballet stance. J Am Podiatr Med Assoc 1987;77:484–9.

[31] Zeiko RR, Torg JS, Rachun A. Proximal diaphyseal fracture of the fifth metatarsal: Treatment of fractures and their complications in athletes. Am J Sports Med 1979;7(2):95–101.

[32] Hamilton WG. Stenosing tenosynovitis of the flexor hallucis longus tendon and posterior impingement upon the os trigonum in ballet dancers. Foot Ankle 1982;3(2):74–80.

[33] Marotta JJ, Micheli LJ. Os trigonum impingement in dancers. Am J Sports Med 1992;20(5): 533–6.

[34] Feldenkrais. Awareness through movement. New York: Harper & Row; 1972.

[35] Loosli AR, Herold D. Knee rehabilitation for dancers using a Pilates-based technique. Kinesiology and Medicine for Dance 1990;8:1–12.

[36] Henderson J, Brown SE, Price S, et al. Foot pressures during a common ballet jump in standing and supine positions. Med Probl Perform Art 1993;8(4):123–31.

[37] Solomon R, Micheli LJ, Solomon J, et al. The cost of injuries in a professional ballet company: a three-year perspective. Med Probl Perform Art 1996;11(3):70–1.

[38] Kolettis GJ, Micheli LJ, Klein JD. Release of the flexor hallucis longus tendon in ballet dancers. J Bone Joint Surg Am 1996;78:1386–90.

ELSEVIER
SAUNDERS

Phys Med Rehabil Clin N Am
17 (2006) 813–826

PHYSICAL MEDICINE
AND REHABILITATION
CLINICS OF
NORTH AMERICA

Foot and Ankle Injuries in Dance

Nancy J. Kadel, MD

*Department of Orthopaedics and Sports Medicine, University of Washington, Box 356500,
1959 Northeast Pacific Street, Seattle, WA 98195, USA*

"The instrument through which the dance speaks is also the instrument through which life is lived...the human body." Martha Graham, 1979

Dance is an art that combines athleticism with artistry. The demands placed on dancers' lower extremities leave them at risk for musculoskeletal injuries. Previous studies have reported injury incidence rates of 67% to 95% among professional ballet dancers and 17% to 24% in modern dancers [1–6]. The foot and ankle of a dancer are particularly vulnerable to injury and represent 34% to 62% of all injuries reported [1–6]. Female ballet dancers have a higher incidence of foot and ankle injuries than male ballet dancers or modern dancers, in part because they dance sur les pointes. In professional musical theater dancers, foot and ankle injuries have been reported as comprising 23% to 45% of all injuries [7–9].

The extreme positions created when dancing on pointe, or on the tips of the toes, or in the demi-pointe position, on the balls of the feet with the ankle plantar flexed, can lead to both acute and overuse injuries of the foot and ankle. Although dancers develop overuse injuries common in other athletes, they are also susceptible to unique injuries. This article reviews common foot and ankle problems seen in dancers and provides some basic diagnosis and treatment strategies.

Types of dance

Today, dance encompasses various techniques and styles such as hip-hop, tap, musical theater, jazz, folk, ethnic, modern, and classical ballet. Although footwear is usually specific to the technique or choreography, most dance shoes rarely include a shock-absorbing sole, and some techniques, such as modern, are performed barefoot.

E-mail address: kadel@u.washington.edu

1047-9651/06/$ - see front matter © 2006 Elsevier Inc. All rights reserved.
doi:10.1016/j.pmr.2006.06.006   *pmr.theclinics.com*

Causes of dance injuries

Anatomic alignment, poor training, technical errors, unfamiliar choreography or style, and environmental factors including flooring surfaces and theater temperature have been implicated as contributing factors to dance injuries. The female athlete triad, amenorrhea, disordered eating, and low bone density, has been implicated in an increased risk of stress fractures in dancers [10–13]. Delayed menarche, common in ballet dancers, has been shown to have an association with increased risk for stress fracture [12].

Rigorous rehearsal schedules, lengthy show runs, and intensive summer dance programs that require an increase in daily class and rehearsal time have been associated with a higher frequency of injuries.

Dancing on pointe

The female ballet dancer often dances in the full pointe position, requiring marked ankle plantar flexion with the toes in a neutral position relative to the longitudinal axis of the foot (Fig. 1). Significant ankle plantar flexion and strength of the intrinsic muscles of the foot and the muscles surrounding the ankle are needed to successfully dance on pointe. The support of the body weight on pointe is borne in the ankle joint along with the tips of the first and second toes. Plantar pressures at the toes on pointe vary with the relative length of the first and second toes and range from 0.14 to 0.58 MPa. When the dancer stands on pointe, the total plantar pressure under the toe box of the pointe shoe is 1.5 MPa. Toe pressures account for 20% to 30% of the total pressure measured at the toe box on pointe [14].

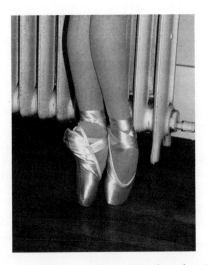

Fig. 1. A dancer on pointe or "sur les pointes."

In pointe work, the stiff shank and hard toe box of the pointe shoe support the foot. In a cadaveric study of sectioning of Lisfranc's ligaments, the stability observed in the pointe shoe demonstrated that the shoe and the closed pack position of the foot in the pointe shoe, share in the remaining 70% to 80% of the load. This supports the hypothesis that the shoe acts as an additional major stabilizer of the foot on pointe [15].

Today's pointe shoes are made from similar materials as their predecessors in the last century. The pointe shoe is composed of layers of paper, glue and fabric such as satin, canvas, or leather [16]. The toe box is initially quite hard, but most pointe shoes are quickly broken in and become soft and pliable with use. A principal dancer may use two to three pairs of pointe shoes during a single performance. Dancers describe poor-fitting pointe shoes that are too soft or worn as dead; dead shoes can contribute to injury.

Turnout

The technique of classical ballet is based in turnout or outward rotation of the legs. Therefore, the movements of classical ballet must be executed in a turned-out position. The ideal turnout demonstrates 180° of external rotation starting at the hips and results in the feet being easily placed in a 180° position on the floor (Fig. 2A). Many students are unable to attain the perfect first or fifth position because of limitations of rotation in the hip, and to place their feet in the correct position, a dancer may resort to pronation or rolling in of the medial arch and ankle, placing increased torque on the medial ankle, tibia, and knee (Fig. 2B). This forced turnout can lead to foot,

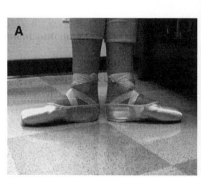
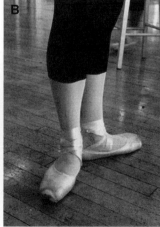

Fig. 2. (*A*) Turnout position of the feet. (*B*) A dancer who is forcing her turnout, resulting in pronation of the medial arch.

ankle, and knee injuries and cause strain on structures around the ankle and knee [17–20].

Metatarsophalangeal joint of the hallux

Hallux valgus

Although hallux valgus deformity is seen in dancers, one study found it was not more frequent than in a similar aged group of nondancers [21]. Dancers with flexible pes planus and those who force their turnout may exacerbate an existing bunion, but dancing on pointe alone does not cause bunion deformities. Young dancers who have hallux valgus often have congenital metatarsus primus varus [19,22].

Bunions in dancers should be managed conservatively. Surgery is reserved only for those dancers who have retired from performing, as any surgical correction may lead to loss of range of motion at the metatarsophalangeal (MTP) joint. Use of horseshoe-type padding over the prominent medial MTP joint, toe spacers between the hallux and second toe, and intrinsic muscle strengthening exercises can help to make dancing on pointe more comfortable for those dancers with bunions [22]. Careful fitting of the pointe shoe, with a higher vamp to better support the hallux MTP joint may reduce symptoms. Emphasis on proper alignment during training of young dancers can help to avoid exacerbation of bunion-prone feet (Fig. 3).

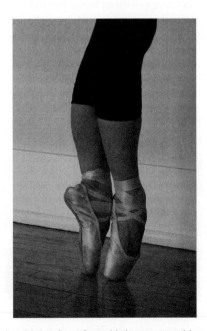

Fig. 3. A dancer rolling in with her front foot; this incorrect position can exacerbate a bunion deformity.

Hallux rigidus

Hallux rigidus is an arthritic condition of the metatarsophalangeal joint. Dancers require 80° to 100° of dorsiflexion when performing relevé onto demi-pointe; therefore, this condition is quite disabling for a dancer. The stiffness in the joint causes the dancer to roll onto the lateral metatarsals in improper alignment or sickling when rising to demi-pointe.

Dancers with this condition report stiffness and pain of the first MTP joint. Dorsal fullness and a palpable osteophyte may be present, and limited dorsiflexion of the hallux. Radiographs reveal joint space narrowing or sub-chondral sclerosis, and dorsal osteophytes depending on the stage of the condition.

Early cases with stiffness, but few radiographic changes, should be treated with gentle traction, passive and active exercises that strengthen the intrinsic muscles of the foot. The dancer should avoid forcing the three-quarter pointe position, as this can exacerbate symptoms.

Surgical cheilectomy with resection of the dorsal one third of the joint, including the osteophytes, can improve symptoms, but as this is a degenerative condition of the joint, the dancer must be warned that surgery will not restore normal function. Recovery time may be as long as 3 to 6 months, and despite a technically successful surgery, some dancers will not achieve the required range of motion of the great toe. Unfortunately, these dancers often have to retire from performing [17–19,22].

Sesamoid injuries

Sesamoid injuries are difficult problems seen in the dancer. Sesamoiditis, bursitis, osteonecrosis, osteoarthritis, and stress fractures are included in the differential diagnosis of plantar MTP joint pain [22]. Prolonged disability can result from these injuries. The sesamoids are small bones imbedded in the flexor hallucis brevis (FHB) tendons, and they articulate with the plantar aspect of the first metatarsal head. They are exposed to significant force when rolling through the foot onto demi-pointe or full pointe and in jump landings. Technical errors such as rolling in, pronation, or forcing turnout can cause excessive loading of the sesamoids, and these should be addressed primarily. Improper jump landings and walking with an out-toe-ing gait also can contribute to sesamoid disorders, as can hip and sacro–iliac joint dysfunction [20].

The presenting symptoms are pain in the plantar forefoot under the first metatarsal head. Tenderness is present with palpation of the sesamoid; the medial sesamoid is most involved commonly. On dorsiflexion of the hallux, the sesamoids move distally, as does the tenderness.

The bursa under the sesamoids can become swollen and inflamed, resulting in bursitis, usually palpable on physical examination. An injection of a small amount of local anesthetic will confirm the diagnosis. Bone scan and MRI may be needed to identify stress fractures or osteonecrosis. Plain radiographs or CT scans can identity osteoarthritis. Bipartite sesamoids are common, but rounded edges seen on a radiograph help to distinguish this from the sharply defined edges of an acute sesamoid fracture.

Treatment includes assessing and correcting alignment and technical problems. Sesamoid pads can be used to off-load the area, and use of a stiff-soled shoe such as a clog or hiking boot outside of class to limit MTP joint motion may be helpful. A removable cast boot may be used if symptoms are severe. Corticosteroid injections in this area should be used only after technical errors are addressed. Sesamoid problems may take months to fully resolve, and need for surgical excision is rare.

Metatarsals

Fifth metatarsal fractures

Missed landings from jumps and rolling over the outer border of the foot while on demi-pointe are two common mechanisms seen in dancers sustaining fifth metatarsal fractures. Lateral foot pain, tenderness, swelling, and ecchymosis are seen commonly in patients with these fractures. Usually the dancer can bear weight, albeit with pain. Physical examination will reveal tenderness over the metatarsal, but radiographs are needed for accurate diagnosis. Treatment for fracture of the fifth metatarsal is based on the location of the fracture. Oblique spiral shaft fractures, known as a dancer's fracture can be treated without surgery even when displaced [22,23] (Fig. 4). A removable cast boot or similar immobilization is used until

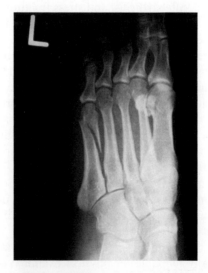

Fig. 4. A "dancer's fracture" of the fifth metatarsal.

pain-free walking, usually 6 weeks. Pool exercises or gentle active range of motion exercises are begun out of the boot as soon as comfort allows. Return to class and performance is done gradually along with a physical therapy program emphasizing proprioception and strength training. The clinician should be careful to evaluate the ankle for instability or injury to the lateral ligaments, as both injuries may occur with this mechanism.

Avulsion fractures of the proximal fifth metatarsal are associated with an inversion injury and lateral ankle sprain. The fracture line is through the tuberosity and is usually extra-articular. These fractures are treated symptomatically, with a stiff-soled shoe or removable cast boot. Surgical treatment is reserved for the unusual case of significant displacement or articular involvement.

Jones fractures occur at the metaphyseal–diaphyseal junction of the fifth metatarsal. They are transverse, and because of poor blood supply in this area, they have a propensity for nonunion. These fractures are more common in modern dancers. Jones fractures can be treated in a short-leg cast for 6 to 8 weeks if the patient can avoid bearing weight, but in high-level dancers surgical treatment may be chosen to avoid prolonged immobilization.

Stress fractures of the proximal fifth metatarsal diaphysis are seen most commonly with repetitive adduction forces such as cutting or pivoting, again more common in modern dancers. The dancer may report a low level of chronic lateral foot pain followed by an acute event. Radiographs demonstrate cortical thickening, periosteal reaction, and a wider fracture line than the acute Jones fracture. These fractures require operative internal fixation, often with bone grafting, as healing potential is poor just as in the acute Jones fracture [20,22].

Stress fractures of the metatarsals

Repetitive loading of bone causes bony stress reactions. Bone remodeling is impaired when loading is increased too rapidly, weakening the bone and leaving it at risk for stress fracture. The cause of stress fractures is multifactorial; amenorrhea, disordered eating, and osteopenia, the female athlete triad, are felt to contribute to higher rates of stress fracture for female dancers. More hours danced per day (greater than 5 h/d) and amenorrhea (greater than 90 days) have been demonstrated as risk factors for stress fractures in female dancers. Most stress fractures in dancers occur in the metatarsals [13], but they can be found in any bone including the fibula, tibia, spine, and hip [24].

The dancer with a stress fracture presents with pain, initially a dull pain toward the end of class or with specific activities. As symptoms progress, pain can be present at night and with normal walking. The pain usually is not well localized, and the physical examination findings are often unimpressive. Some bony tenderness may be found, but usually no swelling is evident.

Initial radiographs are often normal, and this alone should not be used to rule out a stress fracture. Radionuclide bone scans are sensitive to stress fractures and can be positive only a few days after the injury.

Dancers are susceptible to a unique stress fracture of the base of the second metatarsal that is rare in other athletes [25,26]. Runners will typically sustain a stress fracture in the midshaft or distal aspect of the metatarsal. The second metatarsal is recessed proximally, and the first and second metatarsals bear most of the weight when the dancer is in the demi-pointe or full pointe position. A proximal stress fracture must be differentiated from synovitis of the tarsometatarsal joint. In the midfoot, synovitis of Lisfranc's joints and second metatarsal stress fracture are difficult to distinguish with a bone scan. Therefore, MRI is preferred [27]. Healing time is prolonged in the fracture compared with synovitis; therefore, differentiation is important for managing these injuries. Dancers with synovitis may be able to return to class in as early as 3 weeks. Most dancers with a base of second metatarsal stress fracture can be treated with activity modification for 6 to 8 weeks. Casting is not required if the diagnosis is made promptly. Dancers can maintain conditioning with floor exercises, Pilates, or pool training while avoiding pointe work, jumps, and demi-pointe until healing is completed [22,26].

Midfoot injuries

Injuries to the midfoot in dancers, while rare, can be career-ending. The strong ligaments of the tarsometatarsal joints are required for support of the medial and longitudinal arches of the foot. These injuries can be missed, as radiographic findings are often subtle, and the sprain of the ligaments may not be identified without a weight-bearing anteroposterior film. Comparison films of the opposite foot are helpful in subtle injuries. Radiographs reveal a diastasis between the first and second proximal metatarsal cuneiform joints. Lisfranc's ligament is between the medial cuneiform and the base of the second metatarsal. A piece of bone may be avulsed if the ligament is torn, and it may be seen between the first and second metatarsal bases on radiographs.

The mechanism of injury to Lisfranc's joints in dancers has been reported as either a fall off pointe from the full pointe position, missed jump landings, during spins, or during take-off for a jump with the foot sticking to an irregular floor surface [20,22,28,29]. These injuries occur in plantar flexion, with or without rotation.

Dancers with this injury present with significant swelling and midfoot pain. Plantar ecchymosis is seen in more severe injuries. CT scan may identify fractures of the base of the metatarsals and subtle diastasis. Valgus forefoot stress radiographs can determine instability in subtle cases, and they may require anesthesia to be performed adequately.

Most Lisfranc's injuries require operative fixation, and only a simple sprain with no instability should be treated nonsurgically. Cast immobilization and avoidance of weight-bearing activities for 6 weeks, followed by gradual return to weight bearing and activities are required. Those injuries treated surgically will be immobilized, and weight-bearing activities will be avoided for up to 12 weeks. Recovery is prolonged [20,22].

Cuboid subluxation

Acute cuboid subluxation may occur with ankle sprains. The repetitive motions used rising up to and down from the on pointe position are associated with this injury when it is from overuse. The dancer will complain of lateral midfoot pain and an inability to roll through the foot correctly to achieve demi-pointe or the full pointe position. Some are unable to bear weight in acute injuries. Tenderness is usually on the plantar surface of the cuboid. Mobility of the transverse tarsal joints is diminished compared with the opposite foot. A step-off at the base of the fourth metatarsal may be palpable, as the cuboid typically subluxates toward the plantar aspect of the foot. Treatment requires a manual reduction maneuver or passive mobilization of the rear and midfoot joints [30]. Strapping is used to stabilize the cuboid, and peroneus longus tightness should be addressed, as this is associated with the condition. Dancers may require orthotics for their street shoes to control forefoot valgus if present.

Ankle sprains

Ankle inversion injuries are the most common traumatic injuries in dancers. Improper jump landings and rolling over the lateral aspect of the foot while on demi-pointe are the usual mechanisms of injury. In both cases, the ankle is in plantar flexion. As with other athletes, the dancer's anterior talofibular ligament is the most frequently injured. Previous ankle sprain is the greatest risk factor for ankle sprain injury.

Dancers will complain of swelling and lateral ankle pain. If the dancer is unable to bear weight, a fracture may be present. Any bony tenderness over the ankle or lateral foot should alert the examiner that radiographs are required. If symptoms have not improved in a week, then a CT scan of the ankle and midfoot should be obtained to identify osteochondral fractures of the talus or occult fractures of the tarsal bones.

Most sprains resolve with conservative treatment. In a dancer, conservative treatment entails ice massage, compression, and other techniques to minimize swelling. Severe sprains may require a removable boot for 3 weeks. The boot should be worn for sleeping and walking, but removed for icing and early range-of-motion exercises.

Dancers require full mobility of their hindfoot and midfoot joints to dance on pointe. Proprioception training and peroneal strengthening must be initiated early in the rehabilitation of ankle sprains, with emphasis on attaining full mobility of the subtalar and transverse tarsal joints and the ankle joint.

Studies have evaluated proprioception in dancers. Female dancers showed no difference compared with nondancers in proprioception ability. Dancers who had sustained an ankle sprain had altered sensorimotor control compared with those without prior injury, despite having returned to full-time performing and completing proprioception training. Postural stability was noted to improve during the healing process in dancers who sustained sprains during the study period and received active rehabilitation [31–33].

Ankle impingement syndromes

Anterior impingement

Anterior impingement of the ankle is found in male and female dancers. The dancer may complain of a loss or limited demi-plié, and anterior ankle pain on jump landings. Physical examination findings include anterior ankle tenderness, thickening of the synovium, palpable osteophytes, and limited dorsiflexion compared with the opposite ankle. Pain with passive ankle dorsiflexion while the knee is bent will be present. Radiographs will demonstrate an anterior tibial and or talar neck osteophyte. By the time dancers complain of this problem, it usually cannot be solved with conservative measures. The osteophytes typically are anteromedial, and this condition is more common in dancers with cavus feet. A heel lift may give some relief, but they are tolerated poorly in most dance slippers. Surgical excision of the osteophytes can be done through open or arthroscopic procedures. Return to a full plié position may take 3 to 4 months [17,22,34].

Posterior ankle impingement

Posterior ankle impingement is a painful condition of the posterior ankle, caused by compression of the tissues between the posterior edge of the tibia and the calcaneus when the foot is placed in extreme plantar flexion. Posterior impingement pain in the ankle may be the result of a posterior bony block of an accessory bone of the ankle, the os trigonum, or of a prominent posterior lateral process of the talus (Stieda's process). Fractures of the posterior lateral process of the talus also can cause similar symptoms. This condition is seen most commonly in ballet dancers who dance in on pointe and demi-pointe positions with maximal plantar flexion of the ankle. Pain and tenderness are usually posterior and lateral, behind the peroneal tendons. The affected ankle usually lacks complete plantar flexion, both active and passive, compared with the unaffected ankle [35–38].

Symptoms of posterior ankle impingement include recurrent pain, posterolateral tenderness, and ankle stiffness. Swelling may be present behind the ankle joint just anterior to the Achilles tendon. The symptoms are exacerbated by pointe work, relevés, or by any forced ankle plantar flexion maneuver. Some authors have reported concurrent flexor hallucis longus (FHL) tenosynovitis secondary to an impinging os trigonum in dancers [39]. This can cause posteromedial ankle tenderness and pain with flexion of the great toe against resistance. Crepitus may be palpated behind the medial malleolus with range of motion of the great toe. Triggering of the great toe may be present. Functional hallux rigidus may be present, as demonstrated by a limitation of great toe dorsiflexion with the knee fully extended and the ankle in full dorsiflexion.

Radiographs in maximal plantar flexion, or with the dancer on pointe, can demonstrate a bony block or os trigonum (Fig. 5). MRI is helpful to identify posterior bone edema in the talus and calcaneus, and to identify fluid in the FHL tendon sheath.

Treatment consists initially of limitation of painful activities, including pointe work, and physical therapy to work on mobilization of the ankle joint. Having the dancer sleep with a night splint may help reduce stiffness and synovitis. Surgery to remove the os trigonum or release of the FHL tendon is reserved for those dancers who fail physical therapy and correction of technical errors [35–39]. Some dancers benefit from changing their pointe shoe style and fit to a shoe, such as a half or three-quarter shank that allows the dancer to achieve full pointe position with less compaction of the posterior structures.

Flexor hallucis longus tendinitis

Often called dancer's tendinitis, FHL tendinitis is common in dancers. It has been described in other athletes, but it is seen most frequently in the

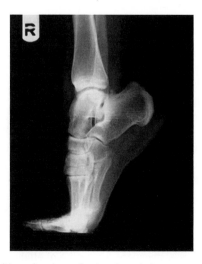

Fig. 5. Demi-pointe position, showing a fractured posterior process of the talus in a dancer with posterior ankle impingement.

female ballet dancer. A biomechanical study demonstrated that the muscles crossing the metatarsophalangeal joints work 2.5 to three times harder than those crossing just the ankle joint in dancers rising on to the full pointe position, placing these muscles and tendons (FHL, flexor digitorum longus [FDL]) at risk for overuse injuries [40]. The repetitive change in foot position from full plantar flexion of the on pointe position to plié with the ankle in dorsiflexion causes the FHL tendon to become inflamed, as it is compressed in its fibro–osseous tunnel along the postero–medial talus under the sustentaculum tali [17,39,41].

Dancers may complain of posteromedial ankle pain, swelling, or popping. Some dancers develop triggering or locking of the great toe if a nodule forms on the tendon. Crepitus can be palpated at the inferomedial ankle, and pain with resisted flexion of the hallux interphalangeal (IP) joint may be present. Functional hallux rigidus may be present, as demonstrated by a limitation of great toe dorsiflexion with the knee fully extended and the ankle in full dorsiflexion.

Conservative treatment including temporary cessation of pointe work and jumps, physical therapy, and anti-inflammatory medication usually resolves the problem. In those dancers with triggering of the hallux or a nodule on the tendon, surgical release may be required [17,19,35,39]. FHL tendinitis may be associated with posterior ankle impingement and an os trigonum, and the posterior bony block can be removed through a medial approach concurrent with release of the FHL sheath in those dancers who fail nonoperative treatment.

Achilles tendon

Chronic Achilles tendinosis may be seen in male and female dancers. Dancers who force their turnout, leading to increased pronation in the midfoot and hindfoot, are at risk for Achilles tendon problems. Failure of the dancer to land with his or her heels on the ground from jumps also can contribute to shortening of the Achilles tendon and risk for injury. Ballet dancers may need adjustment of tight ribbons around the ankle, or the use of ribbons with elastic sewn in the area over the tendon. Careful stretching and the use of a night splint while sleeping can alleviate symptoms. The use of a stretch box in the studio and back stage at the theater has been found to be a good preventative measure for some companies. Acute ruptures are more common in the male dancer, but they can be seen in any dancer involved in jumping steps. Landing in hyper-dorsiflexion or eccentric loading of the foot during push-off can result in an acute Achilles tendon rupture. Acute ruptures in dancers generally are treated with surgical repair [20,22].

> "In a dancer there is a reverence for such forgotten things as the small beautiful bones and their delicate strength." Martha Graham

References

[1] Bronner S, Ojofeitimi S, Rose D. Injuries in a modern dance company—effect of comprehensive management on injury incidence and time loss. Am J Sports Med 2003; 31(3):365–73.

[2] Byhring S, Bø K. Musculoskeletal injuries in the Norwegian national ballet: a prospective cohort study. Scand J Med Sci Sports 2002;12:365–70.

[3] Garrick JG, Requa RK. Ballet injuries: an analysis of epidemiology and financial outcome. Am J Sports Med 1993;21:586–90.

[4] Garrick JG. Early identification of musculoskeletal complaints and injuries among female ballet students. J Dance Med Sci 1999;3(2):80–3.

[5] Nilsson C, Leanderson J, Wykman A, et al. The injury panorama in a Swedish professional ballet company. Knee Surg Sports Traumatol Arthrosc 2001;9:242–6.

[6] Wiesler ER, Hunter DM, Martin DF, et al. Ankle flexibility and injury patterns in dancers. Am J Sports Med 1996;24(6):754–7.

[7] Evans RW, Evans RI, Carvajal S, et al. A survey of injuries among Broadway performers. Am J Public Health 1996;86(1):77–80.

[8] Evans RW, Evans RI, Carvajal S. Survey of injuries among West End performers. Occup Environ Med 1998;55:585–93.

[9] Washington EL. Musculoskeletal injuries in theatrical dancers: site, frequency, and severity. Am J Sports Med 1978;6:75–98.

[10] Lloyd T, Triantafyllou SJ, Baker ER, et al. Women athletes with menstrual irregularity have increased musculoskeletal injuries. Med Sci Sports Exerc 1986;18(4):374–9.

[11] Warren MP, Brooks-Gunn J, Fox RP, et al. Persistent osteopenia in ballet dancers with amenorrhea and delayed menarche despite hormone therapy: a longitudinal study. Fertil Steril 2003;80(2):398–404.

[12] Warren MP, Brooks-Gunn J, Hamilton LH, et al. Scoliosis and fractures in young ballet dancers. Relation to delayed menarche and secondary amenorrhea. N Engl J Med 1986; 314(21):1348–53.

[13] Kadel NJ, Teitz CC, Kronmal RA. Stress fractures in ballet dancers. Am J Sports Med 1992; 20(4):445–9.

[14] Teitz CC, Harrington RM, Wiley H. Pressures on the foot in pointe shoes. Foot Ankle 1985; 5:216–21.

[15] Kadel N, Boenisch M, Teitz C, et al. Stability of Lisfranc's joints in ballet pointe position. Foot Ankle Int 2005;26(5):394–400.

[16] Barringer J, Schlessinger S. The Pointe book: shoes, training & technique. 2nd edition. Hightstown (NJ): Princeton Book Company; 2004.

[17] Quirk R. Common foot and ankle injuries in dance. Orthop Clin North Am 1994;25(1): 123–33.

[18] Khan K, Brown J, Way S, et al. Overuse injuries in classical ballet. Sports Med 1995;19(5): 341–57.

[19] Howse J. Dance technique & injury prevention. 3rd edition. New York: Routledge; 2000.

[20] Macintyre J, Joy E. Foot and ankle injuries in dance. Clin Sports Med 2000;19(2):351–68.

[21] Einarsdottir H, Troell S, Wykman A. Hallux valgus in ballet dancers: A myth? Foot Ankle Int 1995;16(2):92–4.

[22] Hamilton WG, Hamilton LH. Foot and ankle injuries in dancers. In: Mann R, Coughlin M, editors. Surgery of the foot and ankle. 7th edition. St. Louis (MO): Mosby Incorporated; 1999. p. 1225–56.

[23] O'Malley MJ, Hamilton WG, Munyak J. Fractures of the distal shaft of the fifth metatarsal "dancer's fracture." Am J Sports Med 1996;24(2):240–3.

[24] Stretanski MF, Weber GJ. Medical and rehabilitation issues in classical ballet: literature review. Am J Phys Med Rehabil 2002;81:383–91.

[25] Micheli LJ, Sohn RS, Solomon R. Stress fractures of the second metatarsal involving Lis-franc's joint in ballet dancers. A new overuse injury of the foot. J Bone Joint Surg Am 1985;67(9):1372–5.

[26] O'Malley MJ, Hamilton WG, Munyak J, et al. Stress fractures at the base of the second metatarsal in ballet dancers. Foot Ankle Int 1996;17(2):89–94.

[27] Harrington T, Crichton KJ, Anderson IF. Overuse ballet injury to the base of the second metatarsal—a diagnostic problem. Am J Sports Med 1993;21:591–8.

[28] Della Valle CJ, Su E, Nihal A, et al. Acute disruption of the tarsometatarsal (Lisfranc's) joints in a ballet dancer. Journal of Dance Medicine & Science 2000;4(4):128–31.

[29] Kadel N, Donaldson-Fletcher E. Lisfranc's fracture-dislocation in a male ballet dancer dur-ing take-off of a jump: a case report. Journal of Dance Medicine & Science 2004;8(2):56–8.

[30] Marshall P, Hamilton W. Cuboid subluxation in ballet dancers. Am J Sports Med 1992;20: 169–75.

[31] Leanderson J, Eriksson E, Nilsson C, et al. Proprioception in classical ballet dancers- a pro-spective study of the influence of an ankle sprain on proprioception in the ankle joint. Am J Sports Med 1996;24(3):370–4.

[32] Hiller CE, Refshauge KM, Beard DJ. Sensorimotor control is impaired in dancers with func-tional ankle instability. Am J Sports Med 2004;32(1):216–23.

[33] Schmitt H, Kuni B, Sabo D. Influence of professional dance training on peak torque and pro-prioception at the ankle. Clin J Sport Med 2005;15(5):331–9.

[34] Kleiger B. Anterior tibiotalar impingement syndromes in dancers. Foot Ankle 1982;3(2): 69–73.

[35] Hamilton WG, Geppert MJ, Thompson FM. Pain in the posterior aspect of the ankle in dancers. J Bone Joint Surg Am 1996;78(10):1491–500.

[36] Kadel NJ, Micheli LJ, Solomon R. Os trigonum impingement syndrome in dancers. Journal of Dance Medicine & Science 2000;4(3):99–102.

[37] Marotta JJ, Micheli LJ. Os trigonum impingement in dancers. Am J Sports Med 1992;20(5): 533–6.

[38] Kadel NJ. Excision of Os trigonum. Operative Techniques in Orthopaedics 2004;14(1):1–5.

[39] Kolettis GJ, Micheli LJ, Klein JD. Release of the flexor hallucis longus tendon in ballet dancers. J Bone Joint Surg Am 1996;78(9):1386–90.

[40] Dozzi PA, Winter DA. Biomechanical analysis of the foot during rise to full pointe: impli-cations for injuries to the metatarsal-phalangeal joints and shoe redesign. Kinesiology and Med for Dance 1993–94;16(1):1–11.

[41] Sammarco GJ, Cooper PS. Flexor hallucis longus tendon injury in dancers and nondancers. Foot Ankle Int 1998;19:356–62.

ELSEVIER
SAUNDERS

Phys Med Rehabil Clin N Am
17 (2006) 827–842

PHYSICAL MEDICINE
AND REHABILITATION
CLINICS OF
NORTH AMERICA

Repetitive Stress and Strain Injuries: Preventive Exercises for the Musician

Gail A. Shafer-Crane, PhD, OTR, CHT

Division of Structural Biology Colleges of Osteopathic and Human Medicine,
Michigan State University, A514D East Fee Hall, East Lansing, MI 48824, USA

Professional and amateur musicians commonly practice and play their instruments experiencing the physical pain of repetitive stress injury (RSI). Through improved understanding of the etiology and the acceptance of numerous lifestyle changes, including the addition of preventive exercises into the practice routine, the musician may be able to limit the effect of RSI on his or her life. The musician's intrinsic motivation to practice and to repeat motor patterns to perfection compounds the exposure to repetitive trauma [1]. Practice and performance postures are often less than optimal and serve as risk factors for increased RSI. Years, decades, and even centuries of customary practice patterns and schedules preclude the insinuation of ergonomically designed seating and instruments, safer and more comfortable practice methods, and playing positions. Both practice seating and performance seating are often folding or stackable chairs, or flat wooden benches. Lifestyle choices further contribute to higher risk for RSI. Lengthy practice sessions are customary, with short interruptions for fast foods, caffeine, or nicotine breaks. The musician may be unwilling to seek medical help early, because he or she is concerned that the physician will require the limitation of practice or performance times, or worse, instruct the musician to stop playing altogether. In addition, there is a social/work ethic concern about the label of an injured musician [2–5].

On the opposite side of the issue is the knowledge that the most effective treatment of RSI is prevention. Early detection and immediate intervention, within days or weeks of onset, may be effective in most cases for the most complete recovery [3]. Delays in seeking assistance, and delays in the initiation of appropriate care, contribute to severity of the injury and the need for long rest/recovery periods, surgery, or lengthy rehabilitation. Throughout the course of RSI, the musician experiences the loss of practice

---

E-mail address: gail.shafer-crane@radiology.msu.edu

and performance ability, increased pain, and may lose the ability to perform on the instrument of choice completely [3].

Discussing repetitive injury in those whose craft involves precise repetition of motor patterns involves careful consideration, as muscle damage from repetitive trauma is thought to be dose-related. The longer the exposure to an injurious activity, the more likely pain and long-term harm will develop [6]. A phenomenon known as delayed-onset muscle soreness (DOMS) sometimes complicates the ability to notice the early onset of injury [2]. DOMS, well known in sports medicine, also applies to RSI of the musician. Because the onset of muscle pain may be delayed from 2 to 48 hours, the musician may continue playing well beyond the point of injury. As soreness ensues, the musician will adjust playing posture or technique to compensate for this pain. Muscles, tendons, and ligaments unaccustomed to demanding activity are more likely to be injured [2].

Etiology

The literature is replete with repetitive stress injury diagnoses. For the purposes of this article, neurological and muscle diagnoses will be included in the category repetitive stress injury. Other authors have correlated specific diagnoses to the postures and techniques associated with playing specific instruments. These may include repetitive grasping of the strings and neck of the violin, guitar, and cello, which may increase the risk of median and ulnar neuropathies (neurological) or lateral epicondylalgia (muscle). Percussionists are more likely to experience muscular inflammations. Postural requirements, such as supporting the violin with the chin while bowing, may increase risk for thoracic outlet syndrome and neck pain. DeQuervain's tendonitis may be a result of the acute flexion of the thumb for bowing. Balancing on the bench seat of an organ while playing with both hands and feet may contribute to the development of low and thoracic back pain [3–5,7,8].

Localized pain, weakness, cramping, and dystonia characterize muscle injuries. Tendonitis or tenosynovitis, epicondylitis, and focal dystonia are in this group. Muscle damage diagnosed as tendinitis is caused by microhemorrhages, tears at the tendon periosteal junction, and sprains and strains of the proximal tendon [2,6,9]. Extreme fatigue contributes to muscle ischemia and tendon creep [10], increasing the risk of muscle damage. Symptoms generally are localized, and the onset is often traceable to a specific incident.

The etiology of muscle dystonia is understood less well. The pianist is most at risk for this disability involving extra, unintentional movement of the fingers and painful cramping during use [11]. Muscle groups, such as the intrinsic hand muscles and long flexors of the thumb and fingers, contract uncontrollably, resulting in marked flexion of the digits, which is relieved only by discontinuing the activity and redirecting or resting the digits. Pianists are also prone to dystonia of the feet, and trombone players are at risk for dystonia of the facial muscles [8].

There is controversy regarding whether such neural injuries as carpal tunnel syndrome and thoracic outlet syndrome are related to activity. Increased incidence of these diagnoses has been demonstrated to correlate to specific activities [8,12,13]. Neural injuries generally are thought of as nerve entrapments [14–17]. The peripheral nerves pass through muscular and connective tissue compartments as they traverse the distance between the spinal cord and the distant limbs. The nerves must glide throughout their length to limit tension on the individual axons. Connective tissue adhesions limit the excursion of the nerve [18,19]. As adhesions increase, pain may be reported at points along the nerve. This may radiate proximally or distally.

MacKinnon and colleagues have shown that sensory axons in mixed nerves are more vulnerable to injury, because they are located in the fascicles on the periphery of the nerve [18]. Sensory disturbances such as paresthesias, nocturnal numbness and tingling, and hypersensitivity often are reported early in the course of these injuries. As the nerve injury progresses, muscle weakness and atrophy may occur.

Through their course, peripheral nerves travel through sites of common entrapment, including muscular and connective tissue compartments. The prolonged awkward postures of playing many instruments may lead to increased muscle tone and, perhaps, risk of peripheral nerve entrapment. Chronic hypertonicity may result in hypertrophy of these compartmental muscles, compressing the nerves within this more limited space. Further, connective tissue adhesions are more likely, as restrictions within the compartments limit neural glide and blood supply.

Poor posture and subsequent substitution patterns also contribute to compartmental pressure on the nerves [20,21]. Thoracic outlet syndrome is an example of one such injury. Loss of proximal scapular stabilization may lead to rotator cuff tears. Good balance and postural muscle sequencing are essential for proximal stability. Loss of normal muscular sequencing has been implicated in scapular instability [21–25]. Arm pain and weakness are natural consequences of this proximal instability.

Diagnosis

Early accurate diagnosis of a repetitive stress injury is imperative, as is early intervention. Medical history is the number one method of diagnosis. It is important to differentiate between muscle inflammation and neural irritation [26]. Early symptoms in muscle inflammation include localized pain, fatigue, and soreness that may begin during practice, or from 1 to 48 hours afterward. The onset of symptoms may follow a change in frequency or length of rehearsal, a new instrument, different seating, seasonal changes that expose the musician to cold drafts, or a slight injury followed by onset of soreness. Untreated, symptoms may escalate from little effect on either practice or performance, to shortening the tolerated length of practice/performance, to constant pain during practice/performance, and finally to ending practice/performance and affecting activities of daily living [3,5,7,8].

Neural symptoms often have an insidious onset. The irritated nerve defines the distribution of paresthesias. One cardinal sign of carpal tunnel syndrome is paresthesias that occurs at night. Median nerve symptoms include the thumb, index finger, long finger, and radial half of the ring finger. Ulnar nerve symptoms include the ulnar-half of the ring and small fingers. Special tests include Phalen's and Tinel's sign. Although these may be useful, they are not conclusive. Both examination techniques may have false-positives and -negatives [27]. The diagnostic gold standard is the nerve conduction study, which quantifies slowing of the propagation of the neural action potential. Nerve conduction studies require careful interpretation. Carpal tunnel syndrome, for example, continues to be a clinical diagnosis. Combining clinical and electrodiagnositc tests with the medical history is effective in the accurate diagnosis of peripheral nerve injuries [27].

Prevention

The prevalence of RSI in musicians is such that primary treatment for RSI must be prevention. The most effective treatment is education and implementation of healthy lifestyle habits. Good nutrition, hydration, and the avoidance of caffeine, nicotine, and other stimulants are the building blocks of this treatment program. Awareness of muscle fatigue, onset of soreness or mild pain during or shortly after practice, and the will to take frequent rest breaks as soon as these become apparent help prevent RSI [5,7,8]. Aerobic exercise increases peripheral circulation and blood available for neural nutrition. Endurance training, with free weights, elastic bands or tubing, or exercise machines, prepares the musician for long hours of practice and performance, and helps ensure that the muscles and joints are more than up to the stresses and strains required. Endurance exercises can be incorporated into practice sessions. Consistent practice schedules help maintain muscle strength and limit painful overuse. Gradually increasing demands of practice and performance with a new instrument also may limit the risk of overuse injury.

There are many conditioning programs, such as Pilates, Feldenkrais, and yoga. Each is worth implementing as the base of the prevention program. Specific suggestions for exercise prescription will be illustrated [20]. Overall balance maintains the appropriate postural muscle sequencing and enhances core body stability. Prepractice and performance warm-ups are essential. Playing scales or slowly playing simple movements as the practice session begins allows the fingers to prepare for the challenges of playing [7,8]. Stretching has become somewhat controversial. Current research suggests only performing vigorous stretching when the muscles are warmed up to prevent muscle damage from a rebound effect that increases hypertonicity. The exercises should be performed very gently, and within the pain-free range of motion. Postures should be entered slowly, and maintained for 30 to 60 seconds. Long practices should be interrupted by frequent sessions of gently stretching and range-of-motion exercises to improve circulation and relieve fatigue. Care must be taken to avoid pain, bouncing, or forcing the muscles to overstretch [28] (Figs. 1–4).

Movement enhances blood flow through the extremities, relieves fatigue, and bathes joints in synovial fluid. Microbreaks that include range of motion of the neck and extremities at regular short intervals are recommended to help improve comfort, reduce pain, and limit risk of overuse. Gentle stretching programs may be initiated throughout the day, more frequently during practice sessions, and before and following performances. These have some benefit in reducing discomfort and increasing peripheral circulation.

Stretches that have been recommended in numerous websites, textbooks, and journals [7,8,20–23,25,28,29] are simple and gentle. They can be done between sets, and frequently during practice and rehearsal. Note that stretching has been show to be potentially harmful if performed too vigorously, and has not been shown to provide protection from DOMS or RSI [2].

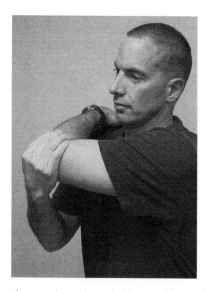

Fig. 1. Each of these stretches may be performed either standing or sitting. In either position, the shoulders are to be positioned in line above the pelvis, the chin tucked in as if trying to make a double chin. One hand is place on the opposite shoulder, and the opposite hand is placed behind the bent elbow to push, gently, stretching the posterior capsule.

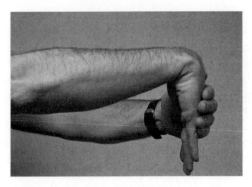

Fig. 2. The arms are flexed to 90°. The wrist of the stretched arm is flexed actively, and then the opposite hand is placed on the back of the first hand to stretch it gently into further flexion.

Ergonomics

Modifications in the instrument, seating, lighting, and even temperature regulation, such as avoiding cold drafts, contribute to effective prevention of overuse injuries. Occupational therapists are trained to assess the individual and match him/her with available adaptive devices. Additionally, they may be able to recommend alterations to instruments [30]. Ergonomically designed seating is available for use while playing specific instruments. Appropriate seating allows the feet to be firmly planted on the floor with the ankles, knees, and hips at a 90° angle. The lumbar lordosis should be supported, and the height of the seat pan requires adjustment that facilitates playing of the instrument. A firm, upholstered seat pan should have sufficient depth to position the musician's back against the back of the chair and the edge, allowing 1 to 2 in clearance to the back of the knees. The edge of the seat pan should be rounded, limiting pressure against the thighs or the back of the knees [31].

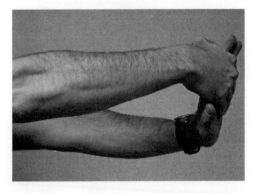

Fig. 3. To stretch the forearm extensors, the stretched arm is extended, and the wrist is extended actively. The opposite hand is placed on the palm perform a gentle stretch to the wrist.

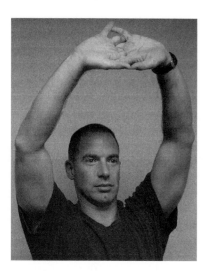

Fig. 4. This is a composite stretch for the shoulders, elbows, wrists, and hands. Starting position is with the fingers interlaced, elbows bent, with the hands resting on the lap. Keeping the fingers interlaced, turn the palms out and extend the elbows. Bring the hands slowly over the head and hold. Return to the resting position slowly.

Treatment and preventive exercises

Early intervention by medical care specialists, such as a physician or occupational or physical therapist, will provide the musician with information about the disorder, ergonomics, healthy lifestyle changes, and an overall exercise regime that may be helpful in stopping the progression of the injury. The initial evaluation takes note of range-of-motion limitations, especially in joints that are more proximal. Poor balance, as in standing on one leg for less than 30 seconds with eyes open or 15 seconds with eyes closed [25], may indicate a sequencing deficit that creates inhibition patterns in postural muscles. Regional strength is tested through grip strength and manual muscle testing. Muscle tone in the neck, upper back, shoulder, and upper limb should be assessed through palpation and manual muscle testing. Hypertonicity in the neck and back supports the notion of a sequencing disorder and suggests the patient may be substituting extremity muscles for posture stabilization over the proximal trunk muscles.

Treatment should include outpatient intervention and a home program. The first intervention includes rest and avoidance of painful activity. Splinting, adaptive techniques, or absolute rest may help to accomplish this. Anti-inflammatory treatments may include heat, ice, massage, counter strain, trigger point release, electrical stimulation, myofascial release, iontophoresis with steroids, ultrasound, or laser therapy. Strengthening of the effected region may follow; however it is essential that the patient be warned to avoid pain. Muscle damage is already present, and working in pain should be avoided to preclude exacerbation of the injury [7,26,32,33]. Emphasis upon trunk posture and scapular stabilization is essential throughout the strengthening phase [20].

Trunk stabilization

One of the elementary exercises for trunk stability is known as the pelvic clock [25]. Patients lie supine with the hips and knees bent to about 45°, feet flat on the surface. They imagine a clock on their abdomen, with the 12 o'clock position toward the head, 6 o'clock toward the feet. Patients then are directed to rock the pelvis toward the 12 and 6 o'clock positions on the imagined clock, using only the abdominal muscles. As patients master this motion, they are instructed to rock the pelvis to point toward each of the hour positions. Patients then are taught the same exercise standing. They stand facing a wall with the feet shoulder-width apart, the hands placed on the wall at shoulder level with the elbows bent slightly (Fig. 5).

Facilitation of the postural muscles and re-establishing normal muscle sequencing for balance and proximal trunk stabilization require gross motor stimulation. Initiation of this treatment is done through balance exercises on a Swiss ball [34–36]. The patient sits on a ball large enough for him or her to sit with the hips, knees, and ankles at a 90° angle. The patient uses abdominal muscles to perform a pelvic clock. As balance is achieved, and

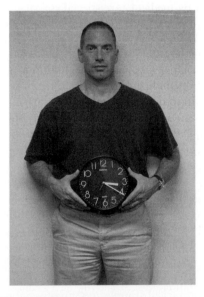

Fig. 5. This illustrates the athletic stance, feet shoulder-width apart, pelvis tucked in a forward pelvic tilt. The illustration of the clock face provides a reference for positioning. The pelvis is rocked in the direction of each of the numerals on the clock face with the abdominal muscles. The instruction to avoid use of the leg muscles for positioning is emphasized.

the patient reports being ready for the next step, the patient is instructed to bounce, making sure maintain at least slight contact with the ball. Balance and coordination exercises escalate, first asking the patient to raise the knees reciprocally every third bounce (hands are on the sides of the ball); then the hands are raised to shoulder level, also in a reciprocal pattern at the same rate. These moves are combined with the patient bouncing, and then raising one knee and the opposite arm reciprocally. Increasing the frequency of the knee and arm raises makes the exercise more complex (Fig. 6).

Shoulder stabilization

Awareness of the position of the scapula during shoulder range-of-motion exercises may assist the patient in establishing improved patterns of shoulder stability [37]. The patient may need to be retrained in engaging latissmus dorsi, levator scapulae, the rhomboids, serratus anterior and posterior, and the rotator cuff muscles in sequence. One exercise that assists with this retraining is the shoulder clock. The patient is placed in side lying position with a pillow that supports the head in a neutral position. The patient keeps the hips perpendicular to the mat throughout the exercise.

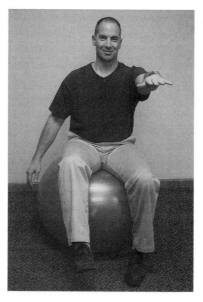

Fig. 6. The weight is centered on the ball. The pelvic clock is an introductory exercise that assists with establishing balance and flexibility on the exercise ball. As balance and comfort improve, bouncing, marching in place, and raising the arms reciprocally are introduced one at a time. These motions are performed in combination as comfort and balance allow. They are made more difficult by increasing speed, height of the limbs in the reciprocal pattern, and complexity of the arm motions. Clapping in rhythm may be introduced as an additional level of difficulty.

The therapist supports the scapula with one hand, while directing the motion of the arm closest to the ceiling with the other. The patient starts with both hands together, arms flexed at the shoulder to 90°, elbows in extension (3 o'clock). The patient is directed to stretch the upper arm so the hand is just past the lower hand. He or she then moves her arm to the 2 o'clock position, and the therapist give feedback regarding the position and stability of the scapula. As the patient moves past the 12 o'clock position, he or she will find it necessary to pivot the upper body so the shoulders are resting on the mat. He or she will pivot back to the original position to complete the circle (Fig. 7).

Upper quadrant strengthening

Shoulder range of motion against gravity is the first step in progressive resistive exercises. Isometric shoulder, elbow, and wrist exercises are added, with emphasis on the musician's ability to limit fatigue or pain by limiting effort. Codman exercises are a widely used program for improving shoulder range of motion. These should be performed early in the strengthening progression with 1 lb weights. As long as the individual is pain-free, low-weight free weight exercises are added and advanced slowly.

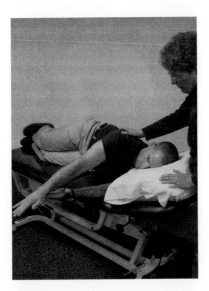

Fig. 7. The shoulder clock is performed while lying on one side. The head is supported in midline on a pillow. The pelvis is maintained in this position throughout the exercise. The therapist manually repositions the scapula, facilitating positions of stability. The free arm is rotated slowly into forward flexion, and the trunk is rotated to allow a full swing of the arm through a full rotation. At each hour on an imaginary clock face, the therapist provides manual feedback to encourage scapular stabilization. After several practices with the therapist, the musician may perform this exercise as part of the exercise regime.

Stress-loading exercises are weight-bearing exercises described as closed chain or weight-bearing. The musician stands next to the exercise ball, bends over slightly bending the knees, places the open hands palm down on the ball about shoulder-width apart. The musician increases the percentage of body weight borne through the extended arms gradually, paying close attention to the position of the scapula reviewed in the arm circle exercise. The exercise is graded by lifting the ball to shoulder height and pushing against the ball just hard enough to maintain its position on the wall. The musician traces a small circle with the ball, moving it by walking hand over hand. As the exercise becomes easier, increase the size of the circle. Finally, when the circles are performed without pain, and can be continued for at least 5 minutes, the pattern is changed from a circle to tracing a large X on the wall. The center of the X is about chest high and at the midline of the body. The ball is rolled up and down along the legs of the X. As the exercise advances in difficulty, the musician must take care to avoid excess fatigue and pain. It may take several weeks to work through each level of the graded activity (Fig. 8).

Upper limb progressive resistive exercises are introduced when the inflammatory pain has subsided [21]. Eccentric strengthening is effective, but if done too aggressively, it increases the risk of inflammation. The progression of the exercise program is initiated with light resistance and low weights. One session is comprised of exercises that use resistance bands, free weights, and exercise putty.

Posture is very important when performing strengthening exercises. The musician is instructed to stand with feet shoulder-width apart, bend the

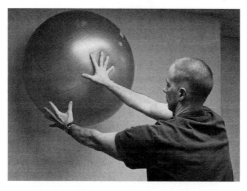

Fig. 8. Stress loading is a weight-bearing activity throughout the upper limb. It is introduced with the Swiss ball on the floor, in front of the musician. The hands are placed on the ball approximately shoulder-width apart, and the weight of the upper body is borne by the hands on the ball. Scapular stabilization is emphasized. The exercise is graded by lifting the ball to shoulder level on a wall, and instructions are given to press the hands into the ball just enough to hold it to the wall. The hands walk it so it traces a small circle. As comfort and strength allow, the circle is enlarged, and finally a large X pattern is traced using the same technique of walking the ball with the hands.

knees slightly, rock the pelvis into the 12 o'clock position, tuck the chin, and adduct the scapulas with arms at the side, a position sometimes referred to as an athletic stance.

Exercise bands made of latex or rubber are graded beginning at very light resistance. There are many brands of these bands, and they are available through medical supply and athletic stores (Figs. 9–11). Each of the exercises is repeated 10 times. The exercises are advanced weekly by increasing the repetitions by sets of 10 up to three sets. Then increase the repetitions to 15. These sessions are performed two to three times a day. Exercises are initiated at 1 lb, and graded up 1 lb at a time to 3 lbs maximum. Emphasis for increasing difficulty is on increasing repetitions.

Exercise putty is one of the products inspired by silly putty. This versatile therapy media strengthens flexion and extension of the hand muscles. Exercises have been designed to strengthen intrinsic muscles and connective tissue structures of the joints. Rolling, pulling, making a donut shape and placing all the digits inside the loop and stretching the fingers and thumb out as if indicating the number five, pinching, and squeezing are among the countless ways to exercise. It is important to limit the length of the exercise. Typically 5-min sessions are assigned, two to three times a day. It is important to stop this and any other exercise at the point of fatigue. No one should be directed to use a tennis ball for strengthening.

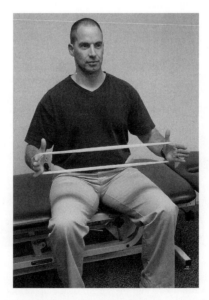

Fig. 9. Loop the band around the back of the hands. The loop is made so it is just long enough so the hands are shoulder-width apart with no tension on the loop with the wrists locked in a neutral position and the elbows at 90° of flexion. The exercise is initiated by spreading the hands apart, as if demonstrating the size of a fish caught, just far enough to be challenging, but not so far as to pull the wrists into flexion.

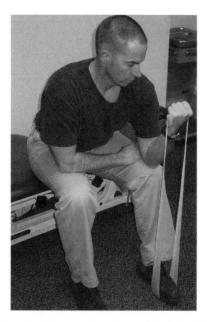

Fig. 10. While seated, chin tucked, loop the band around the ball of the foot; place one elbow on the knee on the same side, grasping the band firmly in the hand with the wrist locked in a neutral position. Perform bicep curls, keeping the wrist locked in a neutral position throughout the exercise.

Neural tension

Neural tension is a significant problem in RSI. As adhesions develop along the length of the peripheral nerve, the nerve is unable to glide through its full excursion. Evidence is noted when there is a complaint of pain or paresthesias in composite range of motion of an extremity, but not during isolated range of motion of a single joint [22,23]. Provocative positions have been defined to evaluate neural tension signs of each peripheral nerve. Paresthesias and pain are the primary complaints. It is possible to use the same positions for treatment. As patients assume the symptomatic position, they are instructed to move in and out of the position that causes the symptom. This maneuver is termed, nerve gliding. It is particularly important for the patient to be instructed to avoid pain, extremes of numbness and tingling, and to be alert for increased paresthesias or pain [7,21,29,38].

Summary

There are many articles that support stretching, strengthening, good nutrition, hydration, rest, and ergonomics along with many other concepts that may be helpful in preventing repetitive stress injuries. The most conclusive literature proposes early recognition of onset of symptoms, and

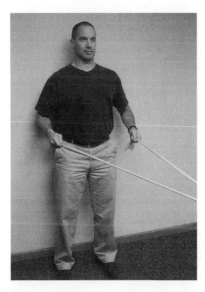

Fig. 11. Resume the standing position after fastening the band to a stable structure, such as the doorknob of a closed door. Grasp the band with both hands; keep the wrists in neutral. Extend the elbows in a rowing motion, bringing them straight down to the side.

immediate reduction or cessation of the causal activity. This is not well accepted by the musician, because this means an interruption of practice and performance. Just like any worker or athlete at risk for RSI, however, the musician must learn to recognize early signs and take the steps to limit damage to muscular and neural tissues. More studies are needed to provide evidence for effective treatment and prevention of RSI.

Acknowledgments

The author expresses her appreciation to Stephanie Shafer for her photography, and Curtis Wood, OTR, CHT, for demonstrating the exercises presented in this article.

References

[1] Brandfonbrener A. Musculoskeletal problems of instrumental musicians. Hand Clin 2003; 19(2):231–9.
[2] Cheung K, Hume P, Maxwell L. Delayed onset muscle soreness: treatment strategies and performance factors. Sports Med 2003;33(2):145–64.
[3] Chong J, Lynden M, Harvey D, et al. Occupational health problems of musicians. Can Fam Physician 1989;35:2341–8.
[4] Fry H. Incidence of overuse syndrome in the symphony orchestra. Med Probl Perform Art 1986;1:51–5.
[5] Fry H. Overuse syndrome of the upper limb in musicians. Med J Aust 1986;144:182–5.

[6] Prasartwuth O, Taylor JL, Gandevia SC. Maximal force, voluntary activation and muscle soreness after eccentric damage to human elbow flexor muscles. J Physiol 2005;567: 337–48.

[7] Norris R. The musician's survival manual: a guide to preventing and treating injuries in instrumentalists. St. Louis (MO): MMB Music Incorporated; 1993.

[8] Safety & Health in Arts Production & Entertainment (SHAPE). Preventing musculoskeletal injury (MSI) for musicians and dancers. Available at: http://www.shape.bc.ca/resources/pdf/msi.pdf. Accessed August 11, 2006.

[9] Slater H, Arendt-Nielsen L, Wright A. Sensory and motor effects of experimental muscle pain in patients with lateral epicondylalgia and controls with delayed onset muscle soreness. Pain 2005;114:118–30.

[10] Maganaris CN. Tensile properties of in vivo human tendinous tissue. Biomed Eng 2003; 31(6):710–7.

[11] Leijnse JNAL. Anatomical factors predisposing to focal dystonia in the musician's hand - principles, Theoretical examples, clinical significance. J Biomech 1997;30(7):659–69.

[12] Personick ME. Brief: types of work injuries associated with lengthy absences from work. Compensation and working conditions online. Available at: www.bls.gov/opub/cwc/1997/fall/brief3.htm. Accessed August 11, 2006.

[13] Stevens J, Witt J, Smith B, Weaver A. The frequency of carpal tunnel syndrome in computer users at a medical facility. Neurology 2001;56(11):1431–2.

[14] Stroller D, Brody GA. The wrist and hand/carpal tunnel syndrome. In: Stroller DW, editor. MRI in orthopedics and sports medicine. 2nd edition. Philadelphia: Lippincott-Raven; 1997. p. 852–963.

[15] Seradge H, Bear C, Bithell D. Preventing carpal tunnel syndrome and cumulative trauma disorder: effect of carpal tunnel decompression exercises. An Oklahoma experience. J Okla State Med Assoc 2000;93(4):150–3.

[16] Rempel D. Musculoskeletal loading and carpal tunnel pressure. Repetitive motion disorders. Rosemont (IL): American Academy of Orthopedic Surgeons; 1995. p. 123–32.

[17] Okutsu I, Hamanaka I, Chiokura Y, et al. Intraneural median nerve pressure in carpal tunnel syndrome. J Hand Surg [Am] 2001;26B(2):155–6.

[18] Mackinnon S, Dellon A. Anatomic investigations of nerves at the wrist: I. Orientation of the motor fascicle of the median nerve in the carpal tunnel. Ann Plast Surg 1988;21: 32–5.

[19] Shafer-Crane GA, Meyer RA, Schlinger MA, et al. Effect of occupational keyboard typing on magnetic resonance imaging of the median nerve in subjects with and without symptoms of carpal tunnel syndrome. Am J Phys Med Rehabil 2005;84(4):258–66.

[20] Liemohn W. Exercise prescription and the back. New York: McGraw-Hill Medical Publishing Division; 2001.

[21] Karageanes SJ. Principles of manual sports medicine. Philadelphia: Lippincott Williams and Wilkins; 2004.

[22] Butler D. Mobilisation of the nervous system. Melbourne (Australia): Churchill Livingstone; 1991.

[23] Butler D. The Sensitive nervous system. Adelaide (Australia): Norgroup Publications; 2000.

[24] Magee D. Orthopedic physical assessment, 4th edition. Philadelphia: W.B. Saunders; 2002.

[25] Greenman P. Principles of manual medicine. 2nd ed. Baltimore (MD): Williams and Wilkins; 1996.

[26] Ranney D. Work-Related chronic injuries of the forearm and hand; their specific diagnosis and management. Ergonomics 1993;36(8):871–80.

[27] Gomes I, Becker J, Ehlers J, et al. Prediction of the neurophysiological diagnosis of carpal tunnel syndrome from the demographic and clinical data. Clin Neurophysiol 2006;117(5): 964–71.

[28] Andersen J. Stretching before and after exercise: effect on muscle soreness and injury risk. J Athl Train 2005;40(3):218–20.

[29] Coppieters M, Bartholomeeusen KE, Stappaerts KH. Incorporating nerve-gliding techniques in the conservative treatment of cubital tunnel syndrome. J Manipulative Physiol Ther 2004;27(9):560–8.

[30] Norris R. Applied ergonomics; adaptive equipment and instrument modification for musicians. Md Med J 1992;42(3):271–5.

[31] Thibodeau P, Melamut SJ. Ergonomics in the electronic library. Bull Med Libr Assoc 1995; 83(3):233–9.

[32] Bottas R, Linnamo V, Nicol C. Repeated maximal eccentric actions causes long-lasting disturbances in movement control. Eur J Appl Physiol 2005;94:62–9.

[33] Nie H, Kawczynski A, Madeleine P. Delayed-onset muscle soreness in neck/shoulder muscles. Eur J Pain 2005;9(6):653–60.

[34] Marshall P, Murphy BA. Core stability exercises on and off a Swiss ball. Arch Phys Med Rehabil 2005;86(2):242–9.

[35] Lehman G, Gordon T, Langley J, et al. Replacing a Swiss ball for an exercise bench causes variable changes in trunk muscle activity during upper limb strength exercises. Dyn Med 2005;4:6.

[36] Lehman G, Hoda W, Oliver S. Trunk muscle activity during bridging exercises on and off a Swiss ball. Chiropr Osteopat 2005;13:14.

[37] Zehr E, Collins DF, Frigon A, et al. Neural control of rhythmic human arm movement: phase dependence and task modulation of Hoffmann reflexes in forearm muscles. J Neurophysiol 2003;89(1):12–21.

[38] Pinar LEA, Ada S, Gungor N. Can we use nerve gliding exercises in women with carpal tunnel syndrome? Adv Ther 2005;22(5):467–75.

ELSEVIER
SAUNDERS

Phys Med Rehabil Clin N Am
17 (2006) 843–852

PHYSICAL MEDICINE
AND REHABILITATION
CLINICS OF
NORTH AMERICA

Upper Extremity Orthotics in Performing Artists

Lawrence L. Prokop, DO

Department of Physical Medicine and Rehabilitation, Michigan State University College of Osteopathic Medicine, B401 West Fee Hall, East Lansing, MI 48824-1316, USA

Performing artists are a special group of patients who place heavy demands on their musculoskeletal structures, acutely and chronically, to pursue their art. It has been said that to miss one day of practice, the artist knows it. To miss two days of practice, the conductor knows it. To miss three days, the audience knows it. This shows the stress that the performer is under constantly to be at the highest level of function. It has also been said that to live is to dance, to dance is to live. This shows the desire that is inherent in many performing artists to continue to perform regardless of the obstacles. Performing is a very important part of their life and often their livelihood. It is also a chronic and recurrent stress on their neurologic, muscular, and skeletal structures.

It is imperative in the medical treatment of these patients that care and concern be directed not only to the diagnosis and treatment of the tissue injured, but also to the needs of the performer. Maintaining a goal of returning the artist to performing as soon as possible will accomplish those goals, as well as improving compliance of the patient. This should decrease the risk of the performer using inappropriate "locker room" remedies as well as the risk of increased impairment if the problem with delayed, inadequate, or partial treatment. Orthotics can aid the entire therapeutic approach to these problems, which includes medications, activity modification, and rehabilitation modalities and therapies.

Diagnostic considerations

Frequently, injuries encountered by performing artists relate to acute and chronic stresses of the performance activities. For instance, we may see tendonitis of the finger flexor tendons and capsulitis of the interphalangeal

---

E-mail address: Lawrence.Prokop@hc.msu.edu

1047-9651/06/$ - see front matter © 2006 Elsevier Inc. All rights reserved.
doi:10.1016/j.pmr.2006.08.002

joints in guitar players, while we see neck and shoulder pain and muscle spasm in violinists. These injuries can be acute when the performer attempts to learn a new technique with difficult biomechanics or performs for longer periods than usual. They may also be chronic when a constant, recurrent activity repetitively irritates and inflames the tissues. Sometimes injuries may progress to significant impairments as the performer may try to stay active with art, ignoring or partially treating the problem. This microtrauma can lead to much worse injury and prolonged recovery, but is usually treatable if addressed early [1].

The examination of the patient should include a history of the problem, how it started and developed, what was done to treat it, what makes it better and worse, and any techniques that affect it. The physical examination should include an inspection of the skin for swelling, erythema, hematoma, and temperature changes. Neurologic examination should include reflex testing and examination for focal dystonia. Musculoskeletal examination should include strength testing, especially of the muscles acting on the hand and fingers, range of motion examination of all joints affected, and examination for discontinuity of joints or tendons and muscle spasm or trigger points. Vascular testing of pulses and vascular compression should be performed. Other physical examination testing should be performed as the history and physical develops. If indicated, testing such as x-rays and electrodiagnostics should be performed. These data aid in fashioning a prescription for the proper orthosis for the patient's needs [1–3].

In an acute injury, the patient commonly exhibits swelling and pain in the area of the injury. Additionally, the patient may complain of pain in a diffuse area extending proximal and distal to the area of injury. Decreased active and passive range of motion often is noted and caused by the swelling and splinting or cocontraction of muscles to decrease painful movement at the area of injury. Swelling may be localized at the site, such as the abductor pollicis longus and extensor pollicis brevis tendons in De Quervain's tenosynovitis, or diffuse as in a myositis or capsulitis involving tendons crossing the joint [1–4].

In a chronic injury, the injured part often is cool as the acute inflammatory response has resolved. Frequently, there is no swelling or there may be a feeling of the tissues being boggy or having a gelatinous coating under the skin. Pain often is present but may be more diffuse and not as specifically located as with acute injuries. The patient may even complain of more pain at other areas of the limb, distal or proximal to the original injury. This may be a secondary effect owing to immobility of the injured limb causing deconditioning, muscle contraction, and joint contracture. There often is decreased range of motion actively and passively. This may relate to the development of joint contractures. There may or may not be splinting of the muscles around the injured part. Trigger points may be noted. Abnormal movements and history might lead to consideration of focal dystonia [1–5].

Tissues affected may be any one in the area of the injury. However, they are most commonly the musculoskeletal and neurologic structures. Muscles may exhibit myositis, spasm, and myofascial trigger points. Ligaments and capsules may show inflammation, contracture formation, or laxity. Tendons may become inflamed and swollen. Nerves may become inflamed and swollen and exhibit pain or decreased sensation or weakness in their distribution. A correct orthosis will aid in treating any of these problems as well as protecting the injured part until it heals.

Treatment considerations

Orthotic treatment for these problems should be in conjunction with the other appropriate treatments and fashioned to the therapeutic and functional needs of the patient. Standard treatment for acute musculoskeletal injuries has been the RICE protocols, where RICE stands for Rest, Ice, Compression, and Elevation. Although this protocol will usually decrease the swelling, erythema, and pain, in the performing artist it may also cause excessive immobility and undue side effects. In this type of patient, therefore, a modification of this protocol is recommended. The new approach is PRICE, or Protection, Relative rest, Ice, Compression, and Elevation. This approach protects the injured area against further injury. Orthotics can restrict the movement to an appropriate range to decrease recurrent overuse and injury and to allow lax ligaments and capsules to shorten and approach a normal distensibility. Use of orthotics to control movement within a controlled range will allow some resting of the joint and allow for decrease in inflammation as well as inhibit the tendency for deconditioning and disuse wasting that can occur with total rest. Ice, compression, and elevation will aid in decreasing pain and the swelling of an acute inflammatory process [1,3,4].

To return the artist to performance as soon as possible, other forms of treatment should be part of the regimen. Pain and inflammation can be controlled with oral nonsteroidal anti-inflammatories, oral steroids, and injectable steroids. If injections of steroids are used, care should be taken to not inject around a tendon or into a joint more than 3 times a year to decrease the risk of weakening the tendon or capsule. In the chronic stage, anti-inflammatories are probably not as effective as in the acute but will often help with the complaints of pain. They may also control recurrent inflammatory response that may occur as the patient works through a rehabilitation therapy program.

Osteopathic manipulative medicine procedures can aid in decreasing muscle spasm by stretching the contracted muscles, relieving swelling by mobilizing fluid, and increasing range of motion by stretching contracted capsules and ligaments. This is especially valuable when the orthosis contributes to muscle contraction and joint contracture as a side effect of immobilization. Therapeutic modalities such as ultrasound scan, paraffin baths, electric muscle stimulation, and others may also aid the treatment at this time by decreasing pain, decreasing muscle spasm, and allowing for greater range of motion with active and passive mobilizations. Chemodenervation with botulinum toxin or motor point blocks with phenol may help the patient who has a focal dystonia [2,4–7].

Orthotic principles

Upper extremity orthotics are used primarily to control movement of the affected part of the limb. This movement control may protect the area from further damage by stopping all movement or by restricting movement to a safe range. Motion control may be needed to correct abnormal postures of a joint such as a contracture or subluxation as well as to assist with movement in a desired range of motion. Although many orthoses have specific names, prescribing by the area of the body they cover is the easiest. Therefore, a wrist–hand orthosis is a WHO. Additional comments may be included in the prescription to include desired functions that the orthosis should accomplish. If the orthosis is needed to progressively increase the wrist extension, the prescription would be WHO with wrist dynamic extension via dial lock or spring extension system. This gives the orthotist or therapist the data needed to manufacture the device to the needs of the patient. Any joint in the upper extremity may have its motion restricted or aided by orthoses, depending on the construction. A static orthosis supports the body part in an immovable position. A dynamic orthosis assists or performs movement in a desired pattern. A major factor in the correct manufacture of an orthosis is 3-point control. The orthosis must stabilize the body part above and below the area to be controlled. These 2 points give the basic structure against which the third point gives a corrective or stabilizing force. Therefore, a static elbow orthosis (EO) will have a stabilizing force with secure structure above and below the elbow. The third point would be the solid area at the elbow itself to maintain the static control desired. At times, the 3-point control is accomplished by a tubular or clam shell structure, which allows forces to be distributed over a larger area: a stabilizing pressure is applied on one side of the limb proximal and distal to the joint, and the counter pressure is on the opposite side of the limb between the two other "points" [1,4,8,9].

In counseling the patient in the need for and use of the orthosis, it is often helpful to inform them that 85% of upper extremity orthoses are temporary. In the case of performing artists, depending on the extent of the problem, the orthosis may only be needed part time, as when not practicing and performing or while asleep. This type of counseling may improve compliance in the use of the device [9].

The benefits of orthoses in the treatment of upper extremity neurologic and musculoskeletal injuries include decreased pain, decreased abnormal range of motion, decreased muscle spasm, and decreased swelling and inflammation. This allows a more rapid rehabilitation and return to practice and performance. In recurrent cases, intermittent use of orthoses may help in controlling the recurrent inflammatory process and pain complaints and thus aid in keeping the performers in their art.

Although the benefits of orthoses are great in this population, the side effects of immobilization may have significant consequences in this population. Neurologic side effects may include decreased balance and coordination and decreased motor activity. Muscular strength and endurance may be decreased. Muscle atrophy may occur. Osteoporosis and atrophy of articular cartilage as well as weakness of ligaments and tendons is possible. Joint ankylosis and fibrosis is a concern. Compression of peripheral nerves and blood vessels has been noted. Pressure ulcers and skin atrophy is also a risk. Although these concerns are most likely rare in this population, they are still a possibility. This possibility highlights the need to make sure the orthoses are fashioned properly so that there is relief over pressure sensitive areas such as bony prominences, superficial nerves, and vascular structures. Prolonged compression of these may cause severe and possibly irreversible damage. The orthoses should be worn only as long as they are needed, and the wearing schedule should be tapered as the patient improves and has less need for the device. As inflammation, pain, and ligamentous laxity improves, the patient should be advanced to an appropriate rehabilitation program. This should include appropriate passive to active range of motion, flexibility exercises, strength and endurance conditioning, and activity-specific conditioning. Wearing schedules should be developed to allow skin tolerance to develop and decrease the risk of pressure sores. A common approach is to allow the patient to wear the orthoses for 2 hours and then remove it to inspect the skin. Any erythema should resolve within 10 minutes. If not, the orthoses should remain off until it does resolve. Then the orthosis is placed back on the patient and maintained for a length of time so that the erythema is resolved within 10 minutes. As the skin tolerance increases, the time for wearing the device is increased [1,10].

A number of materials may be used for orthoses. The body of the orthosis generally is made of a thermoplastic. This allows the therapist or orthotist to shape the brace to the specific patient. It may be lined with padding to decrease pressure and protect the skin. Wrist orthoses often are made of cloth with metal struts or elastic components that restrict movement and are lightweight and relatively cool to wear. Shoulder orthoses are often made of neoprene or elasticized material to aid in compression of the shoulder. Closure of the device is usually with Velcro straps but may use snaps or buckles. Dynamic orthoses may use springs, dial locks, or rubber bands to achieve the force desired. The device must be made so that the forces are directed at the center or rotation of the joint to be moved. If this is not accomplished, then the desired corrective force will not occur or

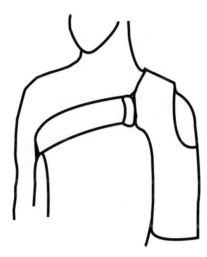

Fig. 1. Shoulder orthosis with arm cuff.

will not be at optimal mechanical advantage requiring a prolonged and possibly unsuccessful treatment.

Orthotics in common use

Shoulder injuries are relatively common. Injuries such as contusions or overuse syndromes of the capsule, tendons, or muscles of the shoulder can be aided by placing the patient in a shoulder orthosis with an arm cuff (Fig. 1) or a sling with or without swath (Fig. 2) to decrease movement and allow for resolution of inflammation. The device is removed easily for

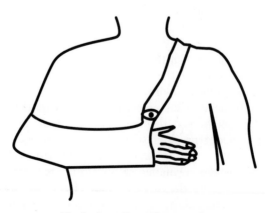

Fig. 2. Arm sling without swath.

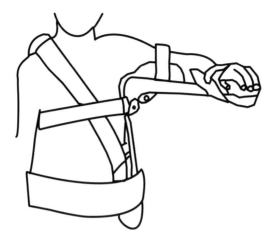

Fig. 3. Airplane splint.

therapy. Because it is not rigid, a modicum of movement in the shoulder is allowed, and this will impede contracture formation. The sling will have a cuff that supports the arm above or at the elbow and a supportive strap system that secures the sling around the neck on the contralateral side. Modifications of this may use straps around the chest or to the opposite shoulder to increase support. If further control is needed, a swath or wide strap wrapping around the sling and the trunk may be added. A special type of shoulder orthosis is an airplane splint. In this modification, the shoulder is maintained at approximately 90°, of abduction and the elbow is maintained at approximately 90° of flexion. The arm and forearm are secured, and struts are connected from the upper extremity section to a support system stabilizing around the upper chest and to the iliac crest. This is used after some shoulder surgeries and manipulations (Fig. 3) [8].

Elbow orthoses may be either static (Fig. 4) or dynamic. There is a proximal support above, and a distal support below the elbow. If immobilization

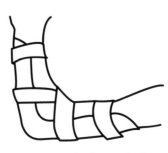

Fig. 4. Static elbow orthosis.

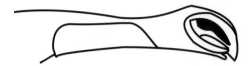

Fig. 5. Wrist hand orthosis with hand in functional position.

or a flexion force is needed, the third point is anterior to the elbow. If an extension force is needed, the third point is posterior to the joint. Static orthoses will often extend around to the medial and lateral aspect of the joint past the axis of rotation to aid in medio-lateral stability. If needed, joints with dynamic spring mechanisms or locking mechanisms may be added at the axis of rotation of the elbow to increase the flexion or extension forces [8].

Wrist and hand orthoses are commonly used as single units. However, the individual components may be fashioned separately, if appropriate for the patient. It is important to remember when using wrist–hand orthoses that contractures may develop. The deleterious effects of these may be mitigated if the hand is kept at close to a functional position. This is 15° to 30° of wrist dorsiflexion, 45° to 60° of metacarpophalangeal flexion, and 10° to 15° of proximal interphalangeal and distal interphalangeal flexion, with the thumb in opposition. (Fig. 5) The orthoses may be fashioned with the major support as a volar or dorsal (Fig. 6) trough covering the distal forearm, extending to the hand and with or without a finger pan as needed. Straps over the interphalangeal (IP) joints, wrist, thumb, and forearm secure the device. Outriggers may be added with springs or rubber bands to increase force at the interphalangeal (IP) joints or wrist to increase the flexion or extension forces (Fig. 7). The force is then delivered through attachments to the fingers

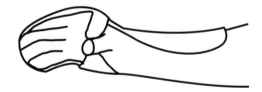

Fig. 6. Dorsal wrist hand orthosis.

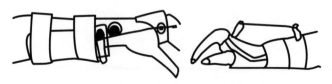

Fig. 7. Dynamic wrist hand orthoses.

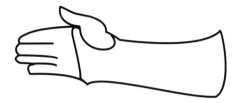

Fig. 8. Wrist hand orthosis without finger pan and thumb section.

or hand to increase the range of motion of the joint desired. These orthoses may be modified as needed. If only wrist control is needed, the finger pan and thumb post may be removed (Fig. 8). If only thumb control is needed, the finger pan and forearm section can be removed leaving only the thumb post and hand section (Fig. 9) [1,8].

Finger orthoses may be either static or dynamic. They come in a variety of styles and shapes. They will stabilize proximal and distal to an IP joint and be secured by fitting snuggly to the individual's finger. Static orthoses will slip over the finger as a ring, a sleeve, or a volar or dorsal splint with support straps (Fig. 10). Dynamic orthoses will have a section at the joint to allow for a hinge mechanism or action with outriggers using spring- or rubber band–loaded devices to increase flexion or extension forces (Fig. 11). Proper fit is required to guarantee optimal forces at the axis of rotation of the IP joint [1,8].

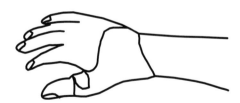

Fig. 9. Thumb orthosis in opposition.

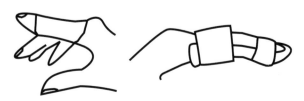

Fig. 10. Static finger orthoses.

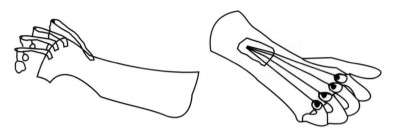

Fig. 11. Wrist hand orthoses with dynamic finger orthoses.

Summary

Performing artists are an interesting group of patients with a need to maintain their activity at as high a functional level as possible. Their injuries generally are acute or chronic musculoskeletal overuse injuries. The underlying pathology of myositis, myofascial pain syndrome, tendonitis, capsulitis, and ligament sprain is essentially the same through the entire limb. The entire treatment of these injuries includes appropriate medications such as nonsteroidal anti-inflammatory drugs, proper therapeutic exercises, training in proper performance technique, and the judicious use of properly designed and manufactured orthoses. When used as part of the whole treatment regimen, these devices will aid in decreasing pain, inflammation, and contracture formation, and aid in improving flexibility, range of motion, and, most importantly, healing time and full return to performance.

References

[1] Tan J. Practical manual of physical medicine and rehabilitation. St. Louis: Mosby Publishing; 1998.
[2] Karageanes S. Principles of manual sports medicine. Philadelphia: Lippincott Williams & Wilkins; 2005.
[3] Mellion M, Walsh WM, Shelton GL. The team physician's handbook. Philadelphia: Hanley & Belfus; 1997.
[4] Braddom R. Handbook of physical medicine & rehabilitation. Philadelphia: Saunders; 2004.
[5] Prokop L. Upper extremity rehabilitation: conditioning and orthotics for the athlete and performing artist. Hand Clin 1990;6(3):517–24.
[6] Greenman P. Principles of manual medicine. 2nd edition. Philadelphia: Lippincott Williams & Wilkins; 1996.
[7] Ward R. Foundations of osteopathic medicine. 2nd edition. Philadelphia: Lippincott Williams & Wilkins; 2003.
[8] Redford J. Orthotics, etc. 3rd edition. Philadelphia: Lippincott Williams & Wilkins; 1986.
[9] Brammer CM, Spires MC. Manual of physical medicine and rehabilitation. Philadelphia: Hanley & Belfus; 2002.
[10] Garrison S. Handbook of physical medicine & rehabilitation. 2nd edition. Philadelphia: Lippincott Williams & Wilkins; 2003.

ELSEVIER
SAUNDERS

Phys Med Rehabil Clin N Am
17 (2006) 853–864

PHYSICAL MEDICINE
AND REHABILITATION
CLINICS OF
NORTH AMERICA

An Osteopathic Approach to Performing Arts Medicine

David Shoup, DO

*Midwestern University of Health Sciences, 19777 North 59th Avenue, Glendale,
AZ 85308, USA*

Osteopathic medicine is a distinctive approach to health care. Andrew Still founded the medical profession over 100 years ago. Still's perspective on medicine was based upon his observation that 19th century medicine was grossly inadequate and sometimes harmful. He developed a new and distinct branch of medicine, which used palpatory examination to find structural causes of medical problems and decreased reliance on surgery and medication. He was more interested in treating the cause rather than the symptoms of disease. His ideas were years ahead of their time and offered a more holistic approach to medicine. In 1892, Still opened the first school of osteopathic medicine, which emphasized anatomy and physiology and osteopathic manipulation. Today, there are thousands of osteopathic physicians throughout the country practicing in all medical specialties.

Osteopathic medicine

Medical education for osteopathic and allopathic students is similar in terms of basic sciences, physical examination, medicine, and surgery. Osteopathic education and medical practice, however, has a distinctive philosophy. The osteopathic philosophy can be summarized in four principles [1]:

- The body is a unit composed of mind, body, and spirit.
- The body is capable of self-healing, self-regulation, and health maintenance.
- Structure and function are interrelated reciprocally.
- Rational treatment is based upon the three statements listed previously.

An osteopathic approach to the performing artist requires attention to these principles. Additionally, the osteopathic education emphasizes

---

E-mail address: dshoup@pol.net

doi:10.1016/j.pmr.2006.07.003

diagnosis and treatment of the musculoskeletal system. Osteopathic manipulation is a hands-on or manual approach used to treat tight muscles and fascia, restriction of joint motion, imbalances in the autonomic nervous system, and decreased circulatory or lymphatic flow.

Osteopathic approach to the performing artist

The incidence of performance-related injuries in musicians, at some point in their career, has been noted to be as high as 70% [2–9]. Traditional medical treatment, including physical or occupational therapy, medications, and surgery, may be beneficial in some performing arts injuries. These interventions, however, may be insufficient for full restoration of health. Performing artists require near perfect function of the musculoskeletal system to meet the high demands of performance.

An osteopathic approach to the performing artist considers all possible causes of the injury and requires a rational, and often, multi-disciplined treatment plan. It may be necessary to use medications, physical therapy, and occasionally surgical procedures. An osteopathic approach, however, also may require behavior or lifestyle modifications, good practice habits, proper nutrition, vitamins and supplements, osteopathic manipulation, and perhaps alternative medicine modalities such as yoga, Tai Chi, deep muscle massage, or rolfing. Osteopathic manipulation is one of the most essential tools an osteopathic physician possesses in the treatment of performing artists. Therefore, an expanded discussion of specific osteopathic manipulative techniques follows.

Osteopathic manipulative techniques

Although many types of osteopathic manipulative technique exist, most osteopathic medical schools teach six common, well-recognized techniques. These techniques can be classified as direct or indirect. Direct techniques require placement of the dysfunctional area of the patient into the barrier of motion (direction of joint restriction or tightness). Indirect techniques place the dysfunctional region into the direction of ease or freedom of motion. Indirect techniques are particularly useful for acute injuries. Common direct techniques include high-velocity low-amplitude, articulatory, soft tissue mobilization, and muscle energy. Common indirect techniques include counterstrain and myofascial release. Other techniques include cranial manipulation, facilitated positional release, the Still's technique, the functional technique, ligamentous articular release, and balanced ligamentous tension.

High-velocity, low-amplitude

High velocity low amplitude (HVLA) involves moving a dysfunctional joint into its restrictive barrier and then adding a short and gentle impulse or thrust through the restrictive barrier to restore physiologic, normal range of motion [1]. Chiropractic manipulation commonly is thought to be this form of manipulation, although chiropractors are skilled in other forms of manipulation also. Even the word manipulation is associated commonly with this technique; however, HVLA is only one of many modalities of manipulation.

In treating the performing artist, HVLA is useful for chronic joint dysfunctions, where restriction of the joint results in pain or lack of mobility. Restriction often is seen in the cervical, thoracic, and lumbar spine of musicians because of the prolonged holding of the instrument and the long periods spent playing in relatively stationary or seated positions. In addition, problems of the wrist and hand are often restrictions of joint motion. Dancers more commonly have joint restrictions and dysfunction of the feet, ankles, and knees. HVLA is applied with care in the extremities.

The steps for performing HVLA are:

- Somatic dysfunction or restriction of motion is diagnosed.
- Soft tissues are treated first to relax them.
- A fulcrum, usually created by the physician's hand, contacts the dysfunctional segment to be treated.
- The dysfunctional segment is positioned to the barrier in multiple planes of motion while maintaining a firm fulcrum.
- Respiratory cooperation or other distracters may be used to help relax the patient.
- An HVLA thrust is delivered against the segment by the physician's hand, thus moving the segment through the pathologic barrier and restoring physiologic motion.
- The segment is returned to neutral, and the motion is reassessed.

Articulatory technique

The articulatory technique involves slowly and repeatedly moving a restricted joint to the barrier of motion (into the direction of restriction). This intervention helps to restore motion in a joint by stretching tight muscles, joint capsules, fascia, and ligaments that may be contributing to joint restriction [1]. This approach is considered a low-velocity, high-amplitude technique (LVHA). Articulatory techniques are especially useful in mobilizing restricted wrist and finger joints in the performing artist.

Soft tissue mobilization

This is used to stretch muscles and fascia. Diagnostic palpation is used to monitor the tissue response and release of restriction. Lateral stretching, linear stretching, deep pressure, traction, and separation of muscle origin and insertion are aspects of this technique. Treatment effects include relaxing hypertonic muscles, stretching passive fascial structures, enhancing circulation, improving local tissue nutrition, and facilitating removal of metabolic wastes [1]. The patient should be as comfortable as possible and remain passive during treatment. Soft tissue mobilization is especially useful for the musician who commonly suffers from muscle tightness in the neck and upper back involving muscles such as the rhomboid and trapezius.

Muscle energy technique

The muscle energy technique (MET) is used to stretch hypertonic muscles. The physician treats the hypertonic muscle by stretching the patient's muscle to the restrictive barrier. Then the patient is asked to exert an isometric counterforce (contraction of a muscle against resistance while maintaining constant muscle length) away from the barrier while the physician holds the patient in the stretched position. Immediately after the contraction, the neuromuscular unit is in a refractory or inhibited state, during which a passive stretch of the muscle may occur to a new restrictive barrier [10]. This process is repeated several times, increasing range of motion of the joint and lengthening of the hypertonic muscle. Performing artists may have muscle hypertonicity in many locations throughout the body. Musicians often have poor flexibility in postural muscles, which can lead to muscle strain and spasm. There may be imbalance between agonist and antagonist muscles because of deconditioning and hypertonicity in opposing muscle groups. This is often caused by a lack of physical exercise and appropriate stretching programs. MET may balance the discrepancy between the inhibited muscles and hypertonic muscles.

The steps for performing MET are:

- A specific diagnosis is made determining the planes of restricted motion.
- The restricted barrier is engaged in all planes, fully stretching the hypertonic muscle.
- The patient is instructed to contract the muscle against the physician's holding force, trying to return to a neutral position.
- The isometric contraction is held for 3 to 5 seconds.
- The patient relaxes for approximately 2 seconds.
- The new barrier is engaged by further stretch of the muscle.
- The process is repeated three to five times. The patient's response is assessed throughout.

Counterstrain

Counterstrain (CS) is an indirect technique that reduces hypertonicity by resetting muscle tone. This is accomplished by facilitating down-regulation of the feedback loop from the spinal cord to the muscle. To treat a muscle in spasm, the patient is placed into the direction of ease or position of comfort. This shortens the muscle that is hypertonic and allows reflex relaxation [11].

It is used often in conjunction with MET to enhance relaxation prior to stretching it. Counterstrain can treat performing artists with acute overuse injuries to help provide immediate relief of pain. This is extremely valuable for performing artists with demanding performance schedules who may not be able to rest for purposes of recovery. Counterstrain is also useful in patients with long-standing chronic muscle hypertonicity that is resistant to stretching and other treatment.

The steps in performing a counterstrain technique are:

- The tenderpoint is located on the patient by firm palpation. Many of these are named according to their location and muscle involvement [11].
- The patient is placed in a position of ease or comfort, whereby the distance between the muscle's origin and insertion is shortened.
- The patient's tenderpoint is palpated with the same firm pressure as the initial assessment. The physician inquires about relative tenderness in the treatment position as compared with the initial tenderness.
- The patient's position is adjusted and fine-tuned until the tenderness is reduced to less than one-third of its initial tenderness (ie, two-thirds improvement in tenderness).
- The tenderpoint is held for at least 90 seconds, with the patient in the position of comfort.
- The patient is returned a neutral position slowly and passively.
- The patient's tenderpoint is retested. The tenderness should be decreased markedly from the initial pain level, thus giving the patient immediate relief of pain.

Myofascial release

Myofascial release treats fascial and other soft tissue restrictions. It can be performed as a direct technique, as in a myofascial stretch. It often is performed as an indirect technique, allowing an unwinding or release of fascial restriction that is restricting motion of the muscle or tissue it envelops. Direct myofascial release simply takes the tissue into the restrictive barrier or in a direction of increased tissue tension and applies forces to stretch the tissue and increase its length. Indirect myofascial release brings the tissue into the direction where it is loose and free of restriction and waiting until the tissue releases tension [1]. This usually requires addressing multiple planes of motion of the tissue such as anterior/posterior translation, clockwise/counterclockwise rotation, superior/inferior translation, and medial/lateral translation. This technique requires a skilled palpatory ability to observe subtle changes in tissue tension. Its use in performing artists extends to any injury in the body. It is especially useful in upper extremity fascial restrictions where loss of efficiency in motion has occurred.

Osteopathic manipulative treatments for common performance related musculoskeletal problems

The choice of the most appropriate osteopathic manipulative treatment for the performing artist depends on the injury and on the expertise of the practitioner. Often, several manipulative modalities are combined to obtain the most efficacious results. There are many osteopathic textbooks that outline manipulative techniques in detail [1,10,11]. The following are examples of the more common problems encountered in the performing artist and osteopathic manipulative treatment for each. This does not serve as an all-inclusive treatment list, but rather a sampling of possible techniques for specific injuries.

Tendinitis or muscle strain of the hand

Musicians, especially string and piano players, are especially susceptible to tendinitis or muscle strain of the hand [8]. Because of the repetitive nature of instrument playing, overuse is common, and recovery is slow. Muscle energy, counterstrain, and myofascial release help to restore muscle and tissue balance and improve joint mobility.

Muscle energy treatment of the hand can be performed on any restricted muscle or joint. The joint is positioned at the restrictive barrier, and muscle energy principles are applied. Counterstrain can be used for treating the muscles of the hand by folding a finger, for example, around a tenderpoint, thereby shortening the muscle, decreasing the distance between origin and insertion, and applying counterstrain principles.

Tendinitis or muscle strain of the forearm

This condition is found commonly in string players in either forearm. Flexor or extensor muscle groups may be strained as a result of repetitive motion. MET may be effective in treating hypertonic muscles, and for medial and lateral epicondyle pain. For example, a wrist that is restricted in extension (or exhibits tight flexor muscles of the forearm) is stretched to the barrier of motion. The patient is instructed to contract his flexor muscles against the physician's holding force (isometric contraction) for 3 to 5 seconds. The patient then relaxes for approximately 2 seconds. Then the physician stretches the wrist to the new extension barrier and repeats the process several more times (Fig. 1).

Additionally, myofascial release can be useful to relax and loosen muscle and fascial restrictions. Direct myofascial release of the forearm is performed by grasping the forearm with one hand at the elbow and the other hand at the wrist. The forearm then is stretched into pronation or supination, holding each position for a minute or two until the tissue begins to release. Other vectors of force, such as a slight traction or compression, may be added at the wrist (Figs. 2, 3).

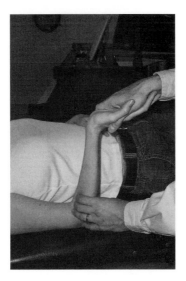

Fig. 1. Muscle energy technique for extension restriction of the wrist.

Shoulder bursitis

This problem often occurs in the right shoulder of string players because of movements of the bowing arm, although it is possible for any performing artist to develop a shoulder injury. One of the most useful osteopathic manipulative treatments for this condition is counterstrain of the subdeltoid

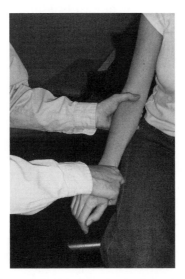

Fig. 2. Direct myofascial release for restriction in pronation.

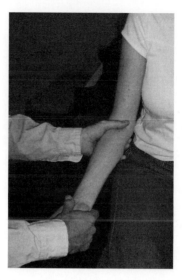

Fig. 3. Direct myofascial release for restriction in supination.

bursa (Fig. 4). The tenderpoint location is found by palpating under the acromion process high on the anterolateral humerus while the arm is abducted slightly. With the patient supine, the physician places the patient's shoulder into 90° of abduction with 30° of forward flexion (the Statue of Liberty position). The position of comfort is fine-tuned with internal or external rotation of the arm. The physician retests the tenderpoint and adds slight modifications in patient position until the patient reports that palpation of the tenderpoint results in at least two-thirds reduction of pain. The arm is held stationary for at least 90 seconds, allowing the tissue to relax under the monitoring finger. The arm is returned passively and slowly to neutral, and the tenderpoint is re-evaluated.

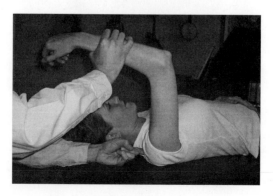

Fig. 4. Subdeltoid bursa counterstrain.

Adhesive capsulitis or impingement of the shoulder

Impingement of the shoulder may be caused by adhesive capsulitis, supraspinatus tendinitis, or shoulder bursitis. These problems often occur from repetitive use following the strain of prolonged playing. Because pain and decreased range of motion are the primary symptoms, myofascial release, counterstrain, and muscle energy techniques are the most useful. Usually abduction and external and internal rotation are limited.

Restriction of shoulder motion can be treated effectively using MET by engaging the barrier of one of the restricted planes of motion. This may cause pain. The technique should be implemented to patient tolerance. To apply MET for restriction in external rotation, the patient's arm is positioned to approximately 90° shoulder abduction with 90° of elbow flexion. The physician supports the patient's wrist and shoulder. The shoulder then is positioned at the external rotation barrier. The patient is instructed to push his or her wrist forward against the physician's holding force (isometric contraction) for 3 to 5 seconds. The patient then relaxes for approximately 2 seconds. Then the physician repositions the shoulder to the next barrier of external rotation and repeats the contraction, relaxation, and stretching process several more times. (Figs. 5, 6).

Muscle strain of the trapezius and supraspinatus muscles

These closely associated muscles are strained commonly in performing artists. For the musician, the holding of the static weight of the instrument or repetitive motions from playing may cause hypertonicity or strain in these

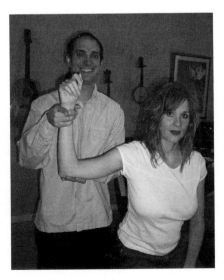

Fig. 5. External rotation restriction.

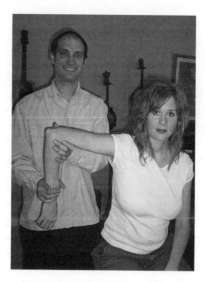

Fig. 6. Internal rotation restriction.

muscles. Following relaxation of the muscle by counterstrain, MET may be used to stretch the muscles and improve range of motion. The trapezius counterstrain tenderpoint location is found by palpating the middle portion of the upper fibers of the trapezius behind the first rib and pressing anteriorly (Fig. 7). With the patient supine, the physician sidebends the patient's head toward the tenderpoint side and abducts the shoulder between 120° and 180°. Follow the last three steps in the example of CS treatment of the subdeltoid bursa.

The supraspinatus counterstrain tenderpoint location is found by palpating the supraspinatus fossa for tenderness (Fig. 8). With the patient supine, the physician adds 45° of flexion, abduction, and external rotation of the

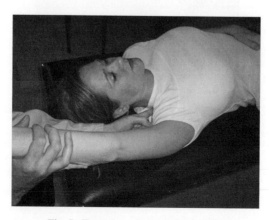

Fig. 7. Trapezius muscle counterstrain.

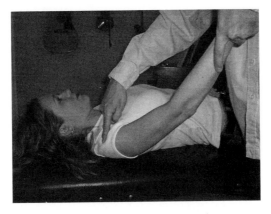

Fig. 8. Supraspinatus counterstrain.

arm. Follow the last three steps in the example for CS treatment of the sub-deltoid bursa.

Neck pain and restriction of motion caused by muscle hypertonicity

Neck pain is a common musculoskeletal complaint in the performing artist. Often this is because of the strain caused from static positioning during long hours of practicing. Violinists and violists in particular may develop neck strain from the static load of their instrument held between the shoulder and chin. Osteopathic techniques are used to restore range of motion of the cervical spine with such techniques as HVLA, CS (used to relax tight muscles), muscle energy technique (used to reduce hypertonicity), and myofascial release (to decrease muscle and fascial restriction).

A simple and effective way of releasing strained muscles and restricted fascia in the cervical spine is by the suboccipital release, a myofascial release technique. With the patient supine and the physician seated at the head of the table, the physician contacts the soft tissue at the base of the occiput with the pads of the fingers. Traction is added in an antero–cephalad direction. As the tissues begin to relax, the pressure continues to be exerted in a cephalad direction. The traction is continued for 1 or 2 min until a release or softening of the suboccipital tissues is obtained (Fig. 9).

Further comments regarding an osteopathic manipulative treatment

Often, there are several musculoskeletal problems coexisting in the performing artist. In other words, muscle spasm in the upper back may lead to muscle strain in the neck and later contribute to tendinitis in the forearm or hand. A single, initial problem may evolve into a more complicated presentation with multiple regions involved. A thorough osteopathic physical examination requires a comprehensive structural examination from head

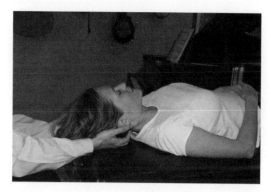

Fig. 9. Suboccipital release.

to toe with emphasis on the area of pain and on other contributory dysfunction.

An osteopathic manipulative treatment usually involves attention to all areas of major dysfunction. This may involve using a combination of osteopathic techniques, requiring meaningful patient interaction. Most osteopathic physicians who specialize in osteopathic manipulation spend at least 30 minutes with their patients. This attention to details is appreciated by the patient and is often necessary to obtain lasting improvement.

References

[1] Ward RC, Hruby RJ, Jerome JA, et al. Foundations for osteopathic medicine. Philadelphia: Lippincott Williams and Wilkins; 2003.
[2] Fishbein M, Middlestadt SE, et al. Medical problems among ICSOM musicians: overview of a national survey. Med Probl Perform Art 1988;3:1.
[3] Middlestadt SE, Fishbein M. The prevalence of severe musculoskeletal problems among male and female symphony orchestra string players. Med Probl Perform Art 1989;4:1.
[4] Fry HJH. Incidence of overuse syndrome in the symphony orchestra. Med Probl Perform Art 1986;1:2.
[5] Fry HJH. Prevalence of overuse (injury) in Australian music schools. Br J Ind Med 1987;44: 35–40.
[6] Caldron PH, Calabrese LH, Clough JD, et al. A survey of musculoskeletal problems encountered in high-level musicians. Med Probl Perform Art 1986;1:4.
[7] Newmark J, Lederman R. Practice doesn't necessarily make perfect: incidence of overuse syndromes in amateur instrumentalists. Med Probl Perform Art 1987;2:4.
[8] Manchester RA. The incidence of hand problems in music students. Med Probl Perform Art 1988;3:1.
[9] Shoup D. Survey of performance related problems among high school and junior high school musicians. Med Probl Perform Art 1995;10:3.
[10] Mitchell F. The muscle energy manual. Volume 1. East Lansing (MI): Met Press; 1995.
[11] Jones L. Jones strain–counterstrain. Boise (ID): Jones Strain–Counterstrain, Incorporated; 1995.

ELSEVIER
SAUNDERS

Phys Med Rehabil Clin N Am
17 (2006) 865–875

PHYSICAL MEDICINE
AND REHABILITATION
CLINICS OF
NORTH AMERICA

Feldenkrais Method, Alexander Technique, and Yoga—Body Awareness Therapy in the Performing Arts

Marcy Schlinger, DO*

Department of Physical Medicine and Rehabilitation, Michigan State University College of Osteopathic Medicine, B401 West Fee Hall, East Lansing, MI 48824, USA

Artistic expression in the performing arts has, at its core, intentional movement. The performing artist executes movement either to create physical, three-dimensional form or to draw sound from an instrument. In dance, mime, or acrobatics, the body itself is the instrument as it responds to gravitational forces. In music, the performer's movement expressly elicits and affects the sound of the instrument. In some situations, the instrument becomes an extension of the body, for example, the bow of the violinist or the drumsticks of the drummer. With voice, the vocal instrument is within the confines of the body, and, therefore is affected by posture, movement, and breath.

For some performing artists, the expression of their craft may be seemingly physically effortless and noninjurious. For many, however, physical limitations may be painful, debilitating, and in some cases, severely disabling. As is evident by the scope of topics covered in this and in other publications, there are commonly recognized patterns of injury and many forms of treatment. There is also increasing awareness of the stresses and injuries to which performing artists are subject.

The purpose of this article is to discuss the Feldenkrais Method, the Alexander Technique and yoga. These three terms refer to complex entities that will be explored separately. Feldenkrais, Alexander Technique and yoga each refer to a highly developed body of thought and theory. They offer the performing artist ways of perceiving and sensing their movement to deepen understanding, maximize function, and at the same time, improve ease and balance. The ultimate goal of all of these is to help the performing artist connect the artistic process with noninjurious integrity of movement.

---

* 4655 Dobie Road, Suite 270, Okemos, MI 48864, USA.
E-mail address: schling2@msu.edu

1047-9651/06/$ - see front matter © 2006 Elsevier Inc. All rights reserved.
doi:10.1016/j.pmr.2006.07.002

Feldenkrais Method

> "The execution of an action by no means proves that we know, even super-ficially, what we are doing or how we are doing it. If we attempt to carry out an action with awareness—that is, to follow it in detail—we soon dis-cover that even the simplest and most common of actions, such as getting up from a chair, is a mystery, and that we have no idea at all how it is done" [1,2].

The original work of Moshe Feldenkrais (1904 to 1984) is the basis for the Feldenkrais Method. Many practitioners throughout the world continue to teach and express his theory. The Feldenkrais Institute in Tel Aviv, Israel, is the repository of his legacy.

Moshe Feldenkrais' life's work is summated as an approach to movement and posture that is conveyed through specific instruction to students in clas-ses or individually or through direct contact in individual sessions. These are identified respectively as awareness through movement (ATM) and func-tional integration (FI). Feldenkrais' knowledge and theory development had a long, circuitous path. At the age of 14, he emigrated, by himself, from a small town in Russia to Palestine. While there, he studied mathemat-ics and worked in map production. Eventually he moved to Paris, where he obtained an engineering degree in mechanics and electricity. He read for a doctorate at the Sorbonne, and during those years, he studied Judo, ob-taining a black belt. He worked in the United Kingdom during World War II as a scientific officer for the British Admiralty. After Israel became a recognized nation, he returned to be the first director of the Electronic De-partment of the Defense Forces. In 1949, his book, Body and Mature Be-havior, was published. From this endeavor and from his experience with knee injuries, his insights about movement, posture, human development, and sensory function led to the development of the Feldenkrais Method [3].

Performing artists may seek treatment with the Feldenkrais Method for in-juries or for preventive reasons. There is no specific prerequisite for treat-ment. Individuals progress through the process at their own rate, and individual benchmarks are developed for evaluation. Effects of treatment in-clude improved flexibility, postural integration, balance, and decreased pain.

One of the tenets of treatment is to examine actions that are complex and to delineate movements or series of movements that are not necessary or are irrelevant to the action. One simple way to think about this is to imagine the violinist who excessively elevates the shoulder of the bowing arm to execute the bow action. The exaggeration of movement of the shoulder in the frontal plane may predispose the musician to pain, fatigue, and muscular imbal-ance. With Feldenkrais treatment, the components of motion are identified to enhance subjective awareness and modification of movement.

Implicit in treatment is the understanding that the global movement of bowing, in this example, involves an infinitesimal complexity of learned and automatic motion. The purpose of treatment is to revisit, with movement awareness, aspects of this process. The treatment helps the artist step away from the automatic patterns embedded after years of practice. The learning process is one of exploration [4]. The process of release and reconnection also may have an impact on the emotional or the psychological state of the performance artist.

Feldenkrais based his theories on his observations and on his understanding of neurodevelopment. He proposed that one's self image is more limited than one's potential capability. Adaptation to and compensation for limitation comes about with movement, intention, and increased awareness. Movement, in fact, is the basis for awareness. In his writings, he addressed habit:

> "A fundamental change in the motor basis within any single integration pattern will break up the cohesion of the whole and thereby leave thought and feeling without anchorage in the patterns of their established routines. In this condition, it is much easier to effect changes in thinking and feeling, for the muscular part through which thinking and feeling reach our awareness has changed and no longer expresses the patterns previously familiar to us. Habit has lost its chief support, that of the muscles, and has become more amenable to change" [1].

In the specific lessons, there is guidance to increase awareness, integrate breathing, increase understanding of the effect of a given action on the rest of the body, and to monitor perception of increased ease and relaxation with repetitions of the action taken. A lesson will describe an action, and then with sequential repetitions advise and instruct the fine-tuning of the action and the gradual, increased range and ease of motion. For the artist–student, awareness evolves from subjective experience and from cueing from the instructor. The artist strives to have more resilience with movement. This comes from playful exploration of movement [4] rather than from achievement in a linear fashion toward a specific goal, for example, trying to increase pronation at the elbow. Even in a group setting, the lessons are individualized as they are practiced and integrated with each person's unique physical signature.

The Feldenkrais Method may be learned in individual treatment sessions or in group lessons. Individual treatment sessions may use FI with verbal instruction and the use of touch to guide movement and awareness. Group sessions use ATM lessons. Feldenkrais teachers are certified after intensive training. The training takes place over 3 or 4 years with over 1000 classroom hours. Resources for Feldenkrais information and training include The Feldenkrais Institute in Tel Aviv, Israel, and the Feldenkrais Guild of North America.

Alexander Technique

The Alexander Technique is a composite of theory and practice that addresses form and function, posture, and movement. The goal of practice is to create ease and freedom with movement or expression. Many theater and music programs teach the Alexander Technique. The history of how Alexander identified the solution to his own voicing dilemma is a telling example of observation and discovery [5].

Australian-born Frederick Matthias Alexander (1869 to 1955) was the originator of the Alexander Technique. At the age of 19, while an actor involved with the recitation of Shakespeare, he experienced recurrent episodes of laryngitis, which did not respond to rest as prescribed by his physician. Aware that his symptoms occurred with recitation, he observed himself in a mirror while speaking. His observation of what he identified as problematic and maladaptive posture led to his extensive lifelong exploration, analysis, and development of theory and practice eventually known as the Alexander Technique.

As with the Feldenkrais Method, the Alexander Technique attempts to help performing artists overcome habitual postures and movements that predispose one to injury or decreased function. Similarly, the mind–body connection is integral to the Alexander approach.

Alexander began teaching his technique to actors in London in 1904. His theoretical construct of the mechanism of primary control is central to his approach. He wrote:

> "I discovered that a certain use of the head in relation to the neck, and of the head and neck in relation to the torso and other parts of the organism...constituted a primary control of the mechanisms as a whole...and that when I interfered with the employment of the primary control of my manner of use, this was always associated with a lowering of the standard of my general functioning" [6].

The use of touch is essential for treatment and instruction. The Alexander teacher, using touch and verbal cues, offers suggestions to the student that correct maladaptive posture and movement and at the same time instruct proper alignment and balance. With treatment, the body is able to access primary control, evoking balance and ease. The Alexander Technique is not specific for a particular artistic expression. Application of the basic principles to any physically manifested action is possible.

In his writings, Alexander referred to the use of the self or good use [7]. These terms imply that an individual may enlist perception and ability for expression in a conscientious and careful way. In his work, he addressed the ways in which poor physical posture and ineffective movement were linked to stress and movement distortion. "Thinking in activity" was another phrase and directive that Alexander used as a guiding principle. Inherent in this concept is the circular feedback communication between action and reaction, posture, and adjustment.

Implementing the Alexander Technique involves a process of somatic reorganization. Alexander instructed students to inhibit patterns through awareness and release of holding tendencies. He also used directives or kinesthetic cues to assist the student in further establishing postural release and a new set point of balance and length. The directives included verbal instructions accompanied by intelligent, guiding touch. "Let the neck be free; allow the head to move forward and up, and allow the back to lengthen and widen" are instructions used by teachers for axial alignment [7].

The official organization (and Web site) for the Alexander Technique is the American Society for the Alexander Technique–AmSat; (http://www.alexandertech.org). The North American Society of Teachers of the Alexander Technique, the American Center for the Alexander Technique, and other national societies also administer teacher training programs and continuing education. The training is extensive; it takes place over several years, incorporating at least 1600 hours of instruction and practice.

Yoga

Aspects of Western society have experienced a remarkable transformation in the past century as Indian and other Asian philosophies and practices have been introduced and absorbed. Yoga and meditation are two such entities. Following introduction, the forms have undergone revision and development to merge with the dominant cultures of the countries of the Western Hemisphere, Europe, and elsewhere.

The word yoga means 'union.' Yoga is one of six classical Hindu schools of thought initially described by Patanjali, sage, philosopher and the author of the yoga–sutra (sutra means thread and refers to a collection of aphorisms or discretely articulated philosophical constructs).

The practice of yoga implies a path of behavior or action taken that eventually leads to a state of transcendence. What is commonly available for many Western students is a practice of yoga that is physically oriented and used for body awareness and conditioning. The philosophy and constructs of yoga in its entirety, however, consist of a complex spiritual, intellectual, and moral set of teachings and guiding principles. The purpose of practice, ultimately, is transcendence of the material world and the confines of the mind. Yogic teachings have their roots in Hindu holy texts such as the Ramayana, an epic tale of the Vedic period, the Mahabarata, (the Bhagavad-Gita is one subtext of the Mahabarata), and the Upanishads (Hindu scriptural texts thought to be the last Vedic revelation) [8].

The traditions and practices of yoga as commonly taught and used include postures (asanas), meditation (dhyana), and breath control (pranayama). Yama (moral discipline) and niyama (restraint) also may be studied and incorporated into practice. These two aspects of yoga, indicative of an ethical foundation, are the first two limbs (anga) of yoga. There are eight limbs in total. Students may be drawn to yoga for many reasons, including the desire for improved physical capability and well-being, and for relaxation and stress reduction. If, in the course of practice, a student delves more deeply into underlying philosophical directives and practice, it will be the result of his or her own investigation or exposure to a teacher who has undertaken an in-depth, continuous study of yoga. The student also may seek out or encounter mystical or esoteric traditions and teachings not as readily available.

According to Miller, yoga was known in Western cultures for many years [9]. Ralph Waldo Emerson and Henry David Thoreau both were interested in the yoga of the Bhagavad Gita. In 1893, Swami Vivekananda, disciple of Ramakrishna, introduced yoga to the World Parliament of Religions in Chicago. In 1899, he founded the New York Vedanta Society (Vedanta–Hindu monistic philosophy). Other practitioners who brought their teachings to Western cultures include T.S. Krishnamacharya, Paramahansa Yogananda, B.K.S. Iyengar, and Swami Satchidananda. In Sanskrit, ananda means bliss, and acarya means teacher or preceptor.

The prevalent yoga that has become commonly available and widespread in the United States and other Western countries is hatha yoga, the practice of postures or asanas. Once obscure, yoga teachers and classes can be found in many communities of varying sizes. The practice of Hatha Yoga offers flexibility, strength, physical resilience, and increased consciousness of breath and movement. Meditation often is taught adjunctively with Hatha Yoga. The practice of meditation allows one to experience silence and a state of serenity and detachment.

Pranayama is the practice of controlling the breath. Prana refers to vital life force. There are specific breathing practices that are taught. Among others, pranayama practices include three-part breathing, a conscientiously monitored filling of the lungs from bottom to top with reversal for exhalation, repetitive rapid breathing with forceful exhalations, and alternating nostril breathing. More experienced students of yoga practice intentional retention of breath. Nadi is the term that refers to energy channels of the body; these are purified and strengthened by pranayama practices. Yoga teaching traditions vary in their approach to and instruction of pranayama. Some use pranayama instruction for all levels of student capability, and others introduce pranayama only after asana practice has been established. In addition, there are more complex practices and instructions for advanced students of yoga.

There are several available schools or traditions of yoga available for students. Specific teacher training programs and methodology are available under the philosophic umbrella of each one. Viniyoga is known as 'yoga for real people' and links breath and movement adapted for individual expression. Iyengar yoga is well known; instruction is focused on precision of form and movement. Bikram yoga is done in greater than 100° heat. Ashtanga yoga also is known as power yoga, with a focus on strength, stamina, and flexibility. Kripalu yoga has central teaching principles of self-awareness and respect for individual capability. Sivananda and integral are two other major forms.

For physicians and other practitioners caring for performing artists, recommendations for yoga will be contingent on community resources, referral patterns, recognition of capable instructors, and communication between colleagues or local information. Although there are many highly respected yoga teacher training programs, training is not regulated or monitored by a mandated professional association. This is in direct contrast to the training for the Feldenkrais Method and Alexander Technique, which are highly organized and internally regulated. Of the three body awareness therapies, yoga is likely to hold the most risk for physical injury.

Students of yoga may sustain injury if they are instructed to hold postures beyond their capability or if a teacher positions them in a way that induces harm. Subtle competition with other students or attempts to do postures without supports or leniency may predispose one to injury. In addition, commonly marketed images of yoga practitioners communicate posture ideals that are not possible for most people to achieve without years of training. The images of yoga–athletes that grace the covers of yoga books, magazines, and calendars convey an ideal more suited to a body building philosophy and may reflect commercial intentions. The images may be superficial or misleading and may be discouraging to students who are otherwise uninformed about the potential for all the positive benefits the practice may offer. Physicians therefore would benefit from becoming oriented in their communities to the resources available and from learning to identify the competent teachers. Yoga teachers, as do many other practitioners, often adapt and change over time; teaching styles and expertise evolve with personal and professional development.

Literature review

There are many case reports and thoughtful, narrative discussions of the three body awareness therapies. Medline literature searches for specific, pertinent research revealed two randomized controlled trials with the Feldenkrais Method as an intervention, two for the Alexander Technique, and 71 for yoga.

In a randomized trial, Stallibrass and colleagues evaluated the Alexander Technique as one treatment arm for a group of patients with Parkinson's disease [10]. The two other treatment groups in the study received massage and no intervention. This is the first rigorous trial for the Alexander Technique published. Outcome measures were the Self-Assessment Parkinson's Disease Disability Scale (SPDDS), a validated scale of Parkinson's-specific disability, reported at best and worst times of the day; the Beck Depression Inventory (BDI); and an Attitudes to Self Scale (ASS). Data collection occurred before intervention, at 12 weeks after the course of intervention and at 6 months. Analysis of the outcome data revealed that compared with the group that received no intervention, the group that received the Alexander Technique had significant improvement on the SPDDS and BDI at the end of the 12-week treatment period. At 6 months follow-up, the Alexander group continued to show improvement on the SPDDS and the ASS and not on the BDI. Compared with the group that received massage, the Alexander group did not have significant changes in scores at the end of 12 weeks. At 6 months, however, there were significant differences in the SPDDS and ASS scores. In the group treated with massage, compared with no intervention, no significant changes were observed. In regards to massage, this intervention has not been compared separately with placebo in other trials. Strengths of this study included a very high compliance and participation rate; 84 of 91 participants were retained throughout.

Ernst and Canter, in a critical review of controlled studies for the Alexander Technique [11], cited an unpublished study by Vickers and colleagues (2000) that evaluated the Alexander Technique in a randomized trial as a treatment arm for chronic mechanical low back pain. The other interventions were 10 weekly self-help sessions or no treatment other than previously established medical care. Outcome measures included inappropriate pain behavior, disability scores, and a pain visual analog scale measured at 10 weeks, and 3, 6, and 12 months. Of 91 subjects, 46 responses were collected at the end of 12 months, revealing no significant changes in the Alexander group. Two other studies, reported by Dennis [12] and by Austin and Ausubel [13], evaluated the Alexander Technique on functional reach and respiratory function respectively. Both studies revealed significant changes in the treatment groups. Limitations, however, including small sample size, nonrandomization of subjects, and lack of control for placebo effects, do not allow for confident interpretation of results.

Johnson and colleagues compared the effects of a course of the Feldenkrais Method in a group of patients with multiple sclerosis with a control group who received sham sessions in a cross-over design study [14]. The only significant outcome differences were with perceived stress and lowered anxiety; other outcome measures that did not show a difference in response were the Nine-Hole Pegboard Test, Hospital Anxiety and Depression Scale, Multiple Sclerosis (MS) Self-Efficacy Scale, MS Symptom Inventory, MS performance scales, and the perceived stress scale. There were, however, nonsignificant trends toward higher self-efficacy after both Feldenkrais and sham sessions. Malmgren-Olsson and Branholm compared the Feldenkrais Method, Body Awareness Therapy, and conventional physiotherapy as interventions for three groups of subjects with nonspecific musculoskeletal disorders [15]. Body Awareness Therapy and the Feldenkrais Method tended to improve health-related quality-of-life and self-efficacy scores over physiotherapy; statistically significant changes were not evident. Ives, in a critical review of existing literature about the Feldenkrais Method, suggests that self-regulation theory, which describes goal identification and integration for change, may be a useful framework for research versus the use of kinesthetic models and motor performance measures [16].

A Medline search on randomized controlled trials on yoga identified 71 studies. There are no specific controlled trials of yoga with performing artists as a treatment group. Several clinically pertinent studies evaluating the intervention and effect of yoga in other populations are reviewed.

Sherman and colleagues compared yoga, conventional exercise, and a self-care book for patients as interventions for chronic low back pain [17]. One hundred and one patients with uncomplicated back pain were assigned randomly to the previously mentioned treatment groups for 12 weeks of intervention (one session per week). Outcome measures were collected by telephone interview at 6, 12, and 26 weeks after the initiation of the study. The primary outcome measure was the Roland Disability Scale; secondary measures were the Short Form-36 Health Survey, degree of restricted activity (determined by responses to investigator questions), and medication use. Practice logs and questions about home practice also were used. Throughout the study, the Roland disability score decreased for all three groups. At 12 weeks, however, compared with the exercise and book groups, the yoga group had the most improvement with back-related function. At 26 weeks, the yoga group continued to have significant improvement for back-related function and with symptom intensity as compared with the book group.

Donohue and colleagues compared the effects of yoga with motivational shouting in 90 high school long distance runners [18]. A third group was a control group that participated in an attention activity of answering several questions. Motivational shouting, compared with yoga and the attention activity was most effective in improving performance on a 1-mile run. Yoga was found to be more effective than the attention activity. Williams and colleagues compared the effects of Iyengar Yoga to an educational activity for chronic back pain in two randomized groups that received the assigned intervention for 16 weeks. [19] The primary outcome assessed was functional disability; secondary outcomes included pain intensity, use of pain medication, pain-related attitudes and behaviors, and spinal range of motion. At the end of treatment and at 3-month follow up, pain intensity, functional disability, and medication use were decreased significantly in the yoga group. Limitations of this study include selection bias (subjects were self-referred) and loss to intervention and follow-up; 70% of those initially enrolled completed the study.

Several meta-analysis reviews have reviewed the effects of yoga on anxiety, breath retraining in asthma, hypertension, depression, and carpal tunnel syndrome. Although these note treatment effects with yoga, study groups often have been small, and methodological errors have made it difficult to draw firm conclusions [20–24].

Summary

The three disciplines described are practiced by many individuals for a myriad of reasons. Depending upon ability and depth of study, teachers of all three disciplines may have specific competencies with which to analyze, instruct, and interact with students/clients. In the author's experience, persons who seek out these practices and incorporate them into their daily lives and expressions of physical activity often are motivated to maintain or establish an optimal state of well-being and function. Physicians and therapists who work with performing artists are in a position to encourage such positive direction in patients, provide information on local resources, and consider the practices as collaborative and adjunctive to medical care.

Acknowledgments

The author would like to thank Judith Barnes, Jeannette Dugan, and Richard Williams of the Chi Medical Library at the Ingham Regional Medical Center, Lansing, Michigan.

References

[1] Feldenkrais M. Awareness through movement. New York: Harper and Row; 1977.
[2] Wilson FR. The hand: how its use shapes the brain, language, and human culture. New York: Pantheon Books; 1998.
[3] Feldenkrais M. The elusive obvious. Cupertino (CA): Meta Publications; 1981.
[4] Spire M. The Feldenkrais method: an interview with Anat Baniel. Med Probl Perform Art 1989;4(4):159–61.
[5] Rosenthal E. The Alexander technique—what it is and how it works. Work with three musicians. Med Probl Perform Art 1987;2(2):53–7.
[6] Alexander FM. The universal constant in living. New York: Dutton; 1941.
[7] Batson G. Conscious use of the human body in movement: the peripheral neuroanatomic basis of the Alexander technique. Med Probl Perform Art 1996;3–10.
[8] Feuerstein G. The yoga tradition; its history, literature, philosophy and practice. Prescott (AZ): Hohm Press; 1998.
[9] Miller BS. Yoga; discipline of freedom. The yoga sutra attributed to Patanjali. Berkeley (CA): University of California Press; 1995.
[10] Stallibrass C, Sissons P, Chalmers C. Randomized controlled trial of the Alexander technique for idiopathic Parkinson's disease. Clin Rehabil 2002;16:695–708.
[11] Ernst E, Canter PH. The Alexander technique: a systematic review of controlled clinical trials. Forsch Komplementarmed Klass Naturheilkd 2003;10:325–9.
[12] Dennis RJ. Functional reach improvement in normal older women after Alexander technique instruction. J Gerontol 1999;54A(1):M8–11.
[13] Austin JH, Ausubel P. Enhanced respiratory muscular function in normal adults after lessons in proprioceptive musculoskeletal education without exercises. Complementary and Alternative Medicine for Asthma 1992;102:486–90.
[14] Johnson SK, Frederick J, Kaufman M, et al. A controlled investigation of bodywork in multiple sclerosis. J Altern Complement Med 1999;5(3):237–43.
[15] Malmgren-Olsson EB, Branholm IB. A comparison between three physiotherapy approaches with regard to health-related factors in patients with nonspecific musculoskeletal disorders. Disabil Rehabil 2002;24(6):308–17.
[16] Ives J. Comments on "The Feldenkrais method: a dynamic approach to changing motor behavior". Res Q Exerc Sport 2003;74(2):116–23.
[17] Sherman K, Cherkin D, Erro J, et al. Comparing yoga, exercise and a self-care book for chronic low back pain; a randomized controlled trial. Ann Intern Med 2005;143(12): 849–56.

[18] Donohue B, Miller A, Beisecker M, et al. Effects of brief yoga exercises and motivational preparatory interventions in distance runners: results of a controlled trial. Br J Sports Med 2006; 40:60–3.

[19] Williams KA, Petronis J, Smith D, et al. Effect of Iyengar yoga therapy for chronic low back pain. Pain 2005;115:107–17.

[20] Kirkwood G, Rampes H, Tuffrey V, et al. Yoga for anxiety: a systematic review of the research evidence. Br J Sports Med 2005;39(12):884–91.

[21] Ram FS, Holloway EA, Jones PW. Breathing retraining for asthma. Respir Med 2003;97(5): 501–7.

[22] Ernst E. Complementary/alternative medicine for hypertension: a mini-review. Wien Medicine Wochenschr 2005;155:386–91.

[23] Pilkington K, Kirkwood G, Rampes H, et al. Yoga for depression: the research evidence. J Affect Disord 2005;89(1–3):13–24.

[24] Gerritsen AA, de Krom MC, Struijs MA, et al. Conservative treatment options for carpal tunnel syndrome: a systematic review of randomized controlled trials. J Neurol 2002; 249(3):272–80.

Further readings

Fishman L. Yoga in medicine. In: Wainapel S, Fast A, editors. Alternative medicine and rehabilitation. New York: Demos Medical Publishing; 2003. p. 139–73.

Jain S, Janssen K, DeCelle S. Alexander technique and Feldenkrais method: a critical overview. Phys Med Rehabil Clin N Am 2004;15(4):811–25.

Nelson SH. Playing with the entire self: the Feldenkrais method and musicians. Semin Neurol 1989;9(2):97–104.

Pratt RR. Art, dance and music therapy. Phys Med Rehabil Clin N Am 2004;15(4):827–41.

ELSEVIER
SAUNDERS

Phys Med Rehabil Clin N Am
17 (2006) 877–891

PHYSICAL MEDICINE
AND REHABILITATION
CLINICS OF
NORTH AMERICA

Music Education and Performing Arts Medicine: The State of the Alliance

Judith A. Palac, DMA[a,*], David N. Grimshaw, DO[a,b,c]

[a]School of Music, Michigan State University, 102 Music Building,
East Lansing, MI 48824, USA
[b]Department of Osteopathic Manipulative Medicine, Michigan State University College
of Osteopathic Medicine, A348 East Fee Hall, East Lansing, MI 48824, USA
[c]Center for Integrative Medicine of Okemos, 4655 Dobie Road, Suite 270,
Okemos, MI 48864, USA

A graduate-level violinist at a major university school of music visits the student health center's physical therapist with pain in her back related to playing. She tells him, "I have to be sure that my teacher doesn't know that I'm hurting. I want him to keep pushing me just as hard as ever."

While conducting a clinic with a high school string group, a conductor asks the students how many of them hurt at times when they play. Over half of the hands go up. When asked how many hurt every day, one-third of the students raise their hands.

These scenarios are common among musicians of almost every age. As a group, musicians tend to be somewhat disembodied; their awareness of their whole selves extends almost exclusively to the parts involved directly with musical technique. Even though many consider musicians to be small muscle athletes [1,2], it is highly unusual to see a group of beginning musicians working out or warming up on their practice field, or having a trainer present to supervise their movements or their mental performance orientation, as one would in sports. Several questions come to mind. How has this state of things come about? What do musicians know about the mental, spiritual, and physical attributes they bring to music making? What do music teachers teach students about wellness? How can a collaboration of the fields of music education and rehabilitation medicine approach these issues? This article addresses these questions.

* Corresponding author.
E-mail address: palac@msu.edu (J.A. Palac).

Historical perspective

Although treatises on musical technique appeared fairly early in the history of Western music, not until late in the 19th century did they address physiological and biomechanical issues in any systematic way [3]. This coincided with the rise of the virtuoso during the Romantic period. The technical demands put on performers by repertoire, and the instruments designed to handle it, undoubtedly made injury more common and thus more of a concern. In fact, the famous composer Robert Schumann's career as a pianist was cut short by such an injury, perhaps partially because of a machine he invented to strengthen his fingers.

The first text to treat technique as a function of the body was a piano pedagogical treatise written by Otto Ortmann, director of the Peabody Conservatory. He set up a research department at the school and based much of his writing on the most accurate physiological knowledge available at the time [3]. Around the same time, Friedrich Steinhausen, an amateur violinist and physician, also wrote a detailed volume on the biomechanics of the violin bow arm [4]. Although such works are scattered through the first half of the 20th century, most pedagogues based their approaches on personal experience and subjective observations. For example, the great violinist Leopold Auer wrote that all pressure for the bow on the string comes from the wrist and fingers, demonstrating that he was not aware of the kinetic principle of summation of forces [5]. The fact that a performer's perception of how the self produces music is frequently inaccurate [6] creates a pedagogical paradox for teachers and students that, if unsolved, produces a fertile ground for injury.

With the explosion of knowledge that occurred in the movement sciences in the 1960s and 1970s, and the evolution of the subspecialty of sports medicine, there was a trickle of renewed interest among some musicians and music educators in the kinesiological and biomechanical issues involved in music making, although it was not nearly as strong as that in physical education. Rainbow decried the lack of research in "objective knowledge of what transpires mentally and physically when a person performs on an instrument" [6]. A few heeded the call. Rolland, for example, conducted a 4-year study on the development of biomechanically sound group string teaching materials at the University of Illinois [7]. His work continues to have a profound impact on string pedagogy today. Bouhuys studied respiratory aspects of wind instrument playing, and Kochevitschy produced a respected text, The Art of Piano Playing: A Scientific Approach [3].

In the 1980s, the wide distribution of the International Conference of Symphony and Opera Musicians (ICSOM) study results [8] and the emergence of the subspecialty of performing arts medicine allowed musicians to unmask their health issues. Music trade and practice publications began to run articles on topics such as types of injuries, healthy technique, performance anxiety, and prevention strategies. Voice journals led the way because of the nature of the instrument. Information on body use methods such as the Alexander Technique began to appear. Some publications, such as the International Musician and Flutist's Quarterly, regularly ran columns written by a medical expert. Janet Horvath, cellist with the Minnesota Orchestra, organized the first conference on musicians' health for musicians in 1987 called Playing Less Hurt [9], and large music education associations (Music Teachers National Association, Music Educators National Conference, and the American String Teachers Association) soon followed with workshop sessions at their national conferences.

Despite the interest evident in practice journals and a call for multi-disciplinary study by performing arts health specialists [10], the body of research on musicians' health by musicians remains limited. The field of music education, which employs both quantitative and qualitative research methodology, would seem to be the natural locus for this type of inquiry. There is a perceived resistance in the music education research community, however, to publication of this work. A few studies have been published in the top two journals, Bulletin for the Council of Research in Music Education and Journal of Research in Music Education, but more have been accepted in Medical Problems of Performing Artists, more multi-disciplinary in scope. The Handbook of Research on Music Teaching and Learning contains chapters on issues related to performance health, by a physician and scientist in the first edition [10], and physicians, scientists and a music researcher in the second [11,12], but, only a few of the existing music education studies or treatises were included in either.

Although more musicians and music educators are aware of wellness issues and try to integrate health-promoting behaviors into their practice, pushing the body, mind, and spirit to the limit for the sake of their art is still the norm. Some teachers still recommend that musicians play through the pain, or demand that students practice an arbitrary number of hours daily without regard for their individual goals or limits. Also, a little knowledge can be dangerous. This author has heard many music teachers recommend stretching exercises (provided to them by a health practitioner for a specific problem) to students for whom they are not necessarily appropriate. For example, it is not uncommon for a string teacher to tell a student with hyper mobility issues to squeeze a tennis ball to strengthen the muscles in his or her fingers.

In a similar vein, well-meaning teachers sometimes exceed the limits of their expertise by trying to diagnose and prescribe treatment for students' ills. Often they do not realize the liability of telling a student that he or she probably has tendonitis and should take a nonsteroidal anti-inflammatory drug, or that beta blockers might be useful for his or her performance anxiety. They are usually unaware of the implications of the Health Insurance Portability and Accountability Act for what and with whom they discuss student medical issues. It seems obvious that more consistent guidance and education are necessary.

The imperative for paradigm shift

In 2001, the National Association of Schools of Music (NASM), the accrediting body for all such schools in the United States, added this statement to its general standards for undergraduate and graduate programs in music: "Institutions should assist students in acquiring knowledge from qualified professionals regarding the prevention of performance injuries [13]." Nothing more was specified. Questions remained. What is a qualified professional? How will this knowledge be delivered? Where will it fit in music curriculum?

Kris Chesky, codirector of the Texas Center for Music and Medicine at the University of North Texas, took up the challenge of addressing these questions. He organized the Health Promotion in Schools of Music Conference, presented by the University of North Texas and the Performing Arts Medicine Association, "designed to facilitate the development of health promotion materials suitable for music students attending NASM schools [14]." The event attracted a wide financial support base from the Scott, Grammy, and National Association of Music Merchants Foundations; the National Endowment of the Arts; and the International Foundation for Music Research. Twenty-five music, music education, and related professional organizations—from the Music Educators National Conference to the American Society for the Alexander Technique—partnered with the conference, each sending a representative. Each of the six hundred NASM schools was invited to send a delegate. This event was pivotal in the advancement of wellness education for musicians and in the collaboration of the fields of music and medicine.

Before the actual meeting, four working groups of experts in the areas of greatest musical health concern—hearing conservation, voice care, neuromusculoskeletal health, and mental health—assembled content they judged to be most important for music students. At the same time, a working group of music educators with concerns or knowledge in these four areas articulated the needs of musicians in each area. All gathered to present their recommendations at the conference in September 2004, with the goal of coming to consensus and taking preliminary steps toward creation of curricular materials for national distribution. Following is a summary of the proceedings [15].

The voice committee, chaired by Stephen Mitchell, focused on knowledge students need for vocal injury prevention. Included were the anatomy and physiology of the voice—the structures of sound production and their functional characteristics. Strategies for maintaining good general health and their specific implications for the voice were discussed. The most frequently-seen voice disorders and vocal problems, both organic and functional, were described, with an emphasis on the adverse effects of common medications on vocal health. The committee also gave criteria for resting the voice and for seeking professional care.

The hearing health committee, chaired by Miriam Henoch, developed recommendations for educating music students to avoid irreversible noise-induced hearing loss. The group focused on the anatomy of the ear and the effects of detrimental sound exposure on its structures. The members presented several strategies for protecting hearing. The necessity of using hearing protection devices (earplugs), and the advantages and disadvantages of many different kinds of hearing protection devices, were discussed. The committee also presented the standards for sound exposure developed by the Office of Occupational Safety and Health Administration (OSHA) and gave examples of sound pressures generated in different musical situations, which are often too high for prolonged exposure.

An overview of neuromusculoskeletal health issues was presented by that working group, chaired by Ralph Manchester. Members described various muscle–tendon problems, such as tendonitis, and neurological problems, such as carpal tunnel syndrome, and risk factors for injuries and disorders. Anatomy and physiology of the affected body parts also were discussed. The committee described treatments and suggested preventive strategies. The group also advocated exploration of the patient–doctor relationship.

The mental health working group under the direction of Susan Raeburn recommended issues such as psychological disorders and performance anxiety for inclusion in college music students' study. Members also addressed the effect of stress on musicians' health and performance, and emphasized the importance of the teacher's role in stress inoculation. Information about substance abuse was presented. Challenging career issues, including the scarcity of performance jobs, were discussed as well.

The music education working group, headed by Don Hodges, articulated musicians' educational needs in each of the four content areas. It also dealt with issues of curriculum. Fitting this information in the right place in already overcrowded programs, especially in preservice teacher education, was discussed. The group suggested other avenues of dissemination to the music education profession, such as professional in-services, conferences, and journals. The imperative for multi-disciplinary research on these aspects of music making, and issues surrounding publication of that research, were discussed.

The conference laid a foundation of knowledge that music students need for wellness. Chesky submitted curricular recommendations developed by Health Promotion in Schools of Music to NASM for acceptance in January 2006; they were accepted and are now available to all accredited schools of music [16]. These curricular frameworks and conference proceedings are available on the HPSM Web site.

As Chesky stated in the introduction to the conference,

"Educating college music students about health issues is a daunting task that requires involvement from several disciplines and perspectives. Success will depend on our ability to create and sustain working collaborations that help challenge, redefine, and expand what is currently known and accepted [15]."

The paradigm in music making and teaching is beginning to shift in a healthy direction.

The role of medicine for the musician

As the music education community works to heed the imperative for a paradigm shift toward an educational culture that will help students learn what they need to know to keep themselves healthy, the physical medicine and rehabilitation community can be a valuable resource for this special population of highly trained and motivated artists and educators. With a focus on function and the structure of a team-based approach already in place, physiatric practice is a place where musicians may be able to find the tools and resources they need for the shift to a more embodied approach to education and practice. The lessons needed for the music education culture, however, are needed in medical education also. It is ironic that even the profession entrusted with the task of healing the body is just as disembodied in its methods and practices as other professions [17]. Much time and effort is spent on streamlining guidelines for the treatment of various disorders and the development of procedures that offer a fix for the injured patient, when patients with the same disorder look so very different from one another and require different approaches to achieve the desired result: return to function, return to wholeness.

Where do the needs of musicians and the strengths inherent in an integrative physical medicine and rehabilitation approach intersect? Musicians need to be exceptional communicators, have the capacity and dynamic vitality to perform their work at a high level of ability over time, and depend upon their bodies as the vehicle for the expression of their vocational calling. They need to be in close relationship with and possess detailed understanding of their bodies and the relationship between their thoughts, feelings, and physical functioning. They also need to be able to sustain health over time to remain competent in their field.

An integrative approach to medical practice looks at health as a dynamic state that depends upon the ongoing support and nurturance of the person (mind/body/spirit), which possesses the ability to be self-organizing, and to heal when given the appropriate ingredients and environment. The ingredients can be organized within a conceptual construct that includes physical, emotional, mental, and spiritual elements.

Physical elements

These consist of nutrition, sleep, movement, rhythmic patterns of activity and rest, sunshine, shelter, and protection from harm.

Emotional elements

These include a safe and consistent environment, meaningful relationships, meaningful work that is consistent with beliefs and abilities, community, and reliable access to trustworthy information.

Mental elements

These consist of belief that work is meaningful and contributes to the world, ability to exercise abilities and talents without censure, and creative interactions with others and with ideas.

Spiritual elements

These include an evolving understanding of who a person is, an evolving understanding of who one loves, a sense of purpose, and being able to see how one's contributions fit into a larger scheme that makes sense [18–20].

The role of the arts and of arts education is of paramount importance in the well being of any culture. Modern culture has lost its connection to history, place, and inherent values. A part of both medical and music education that has been omitted because of the current cultural model of reality is the teaching of how one learns to develop, test, and refine the ability to gain subjective knowledge about oneself, especially one's body. Teachers and students lack understanding and experience with how one obtains knowledge and an internal sense of balance, or reliably judges the right relationship of things. Most people progress through tactile, auditory, visual, vestibular, and proprioceptive learning as infants and children without much difficulty. However, the degree to which one is able to achieve higher orders of cognitive, perceptual, and sensorimotor integration as one matures varies considerably between people and is highly important in the performing arts fields. Small losses mean huge impairments to musicians. These elements of the way one experiences, interprets, and integrates senses to function in the world are fundamental health skills. Although these more subjective elements of one's internal state of health are harder to access, understand, and remedy, it remains for people to explore ways of acknowledging their powerful impact on the healing of persons. Medical practice inspires one to look for ways to help patients regain these elements when injury or illness creates disorganization and confusion in their physiological relationships. Motor planning without sensory integration is a lost cause, and yet much time and energy is spent putting the cart before the horse in therapy [21,22].

Case history

The story of a 20-year-old female violinist who sought help for disabling pains in three different regions of her left upper extremity serves to illustrate.

This young woman was at the time of evaluation in her third year of studies at the school of music majoring in performance. She had been playing the violin for 17 years without injury or impairment other than brief episodes of muscular fatigue at times of increased intensity during her high school years. She studied violin according to the Suzuki method beginning at age 3. In addition to regular weekly lessons, she attended several week-long summer institutes over the years, during which she was taught by several different teachers, as is the tradition in the Suzuki approach. She expressed that, by the time she entered college, she observed that she was a stiffer player than many of her peers, but that because no teacher had ever spoken to her about tension in her playing, she assumed that was normal. Once at school, she wondered why everything that she seemed to struggle with looked so easy for other students. She developed wrist pain after she participated in scale boot camp with her teacher and some other students, consisting of several hours a day of intensive technical exercises. Following that, her teacher insisted that she take her shoulder pad off and be willing to play through the pain. He recanted, however, when it was apparent that her pain became worse.

She went to the student health center for advice and help. She was seen by an orthopedic surgeon and then a physical therapist. She received instruction in stretches for wrist, arm, and shoulder, Thera-Band exercises, and upper extremity movement on an ergonomic hand-driven wheel three times a week for 3 weeks. She also took ibuprofen during this time, 800 mg by mouth twice daily.

Unfortunately, her symptoms escalated and expanded during this 3-week course of physical therapy considered appropriate for the disorder. By the latter part of the fall term, she had severe continuous pain in the lateral aspect of her elbow, in the dorsal aspect of her wrist, and in the anterior aspect of her shoulder. This created in her a sense of desperation, as her primary vocational goal and her source of income were being threatened. Her first two attempts to attend to the problem seemed to have backfired. Without previous experience in these matters, she had no reference for what to expect or how to judge her response to treatment. Indeed, she felt her body had failed her when she needed it the most, creating a mind/body disconnect that escalated the intensity of her crisis at the crossroads of health and vocation.

Fortunately, she spoke with a professor knowledgeable about injuries in performing artists and agreed to see another doctor about the problem before giving up. It took a great deal of encouragement to get her to seek further assistance, because her experience had been noxious enough to lead her to contemplate a complete change in career path.

Her past medical history was not significant for any medical problems. She had tonsils and adenoids removed as a child, a broken right foot in high school, and a broken left fifth phalanx in grade school. The fractures had healed without sequelae. She had not experienced any chronic illnesses or infections during childhood. She met normal developmental and academic milestones throughout primary and secondary school years.

She was single, a nonsmoker, did not use alcohol or illicit drugs, lived alone, and did all of her own self-care and homemaking tasks. She averaged two cups of coffee per day; sleep was adequate without difficulty, and she was not overweight or deconditioned. She was right-hand dominant. Her self-image, however, did not include a sense of confidence in her physical abilities or kinesthetic competency.

Medications were ibuprofen 800 mg twice daily. Allergies were NKDA, environmental: dust and ragweed.

Review of systems was negative, except for occasional irregular menses, with dysmenorrhea, and headache usually just before menses. Psychiatric history was negative. Family history showed mother and grandmother with obesity and osteoarthritis of knees.

On examination, she was an alert, articulate young woman of average height. She had normal vital signs and no integumentary lesions. She wore glasses and was Caucasian. She had the ability to perform the elements of a screening neuromusculoskeletal examination without difficulty and with awareness, and she could stand and sit with apparently normal posture. There were only minimal, segmental restrictions in the spine at L4, T4, and T5. The primary findings were pain on palpation at the radial head, lateral epicondyle, biceps tendon at the bicipital groove, levator scapula insertion, and at several points within the upper trapezius, teres major, and upon the dorsal aspect of the distal forearm—all on the left upper extremity. Range of motion was reduced by approximately 15° in supination of the forearm, at the end of range of elbow extension, and in upward rotation and external rotation of the scapulothoracic motions associated with abduction and horizontal abduction of the shoulder. Upper limb tension tests revealed a mildly positive median nerve bias, made moderately positive by adding scapular depression on the left side only [23]. She had some apparent weakness of the anterior deltoid, appearing to be primarily related to pain.

As she played the violin, it was apparent that the pain was affecting her ability to maintain her usual posture, technique, and proficiency. She was visibly cringing with longer passages and bringing her left arm more medially and inferiorly with time. The lack of full supination at the forearm created difficulties for her with fingering, especially in the higher registers.

Initial treatment was to use an injection of procaine and triamcinolone in the regions of the lateral epicondyle and radial head, and manual therapy of myofascial, functional indirect, and muscle energy types to the areas of motion restriction. She and the doctor continued the ibuprofen, and she obtained a new chin rest and shoulder pad for her violin. These measures together allowed some relief, and she and the doctor shifted their focus to a more long-term plan of care. How to prevent this from ever getting this bad again? What seemed most important was to help her address the issues of internal balance/postural awareness and to re-establish movement patterns that would be sustainable over time as a performer.

Convincing her that another trial of physical therapy was worthwhile took some extended dialog. Much thought went into deciding where to send her including knowledge of the experience, skill level, and ability of the chosen therapist to have interactive patience in teaching such things as physiological quieting and kinesthetic awareness. A very specific referral was made to a therapist with performing arts medicine experience and a personality that would allow a much more individualized approach to the problem. In such a case, the environment where care is delivered is also quite important. The context of care needs to be a place where the patient will be heard and given the time and space to literally learn to listen to his or her own body.

As they began, movement patterns of her upper extremity were assessed in the context of cervical, thoracic, clavicular, and scapular motions. As neural glide mobilizations and manual stretching were initiated, it was noted that she had difficulty with both abdominal and scapular stabilization, and a thorough plan of treatment was created for her that included therapeutic exercise detailed as follows:

- Instruction in physiological quieting (diaphragmatic breathing, awareness of movement of pelvis, trunk, and upper quarter stabilizing musculature)
- Stretching of shortened musculature
- Joint mobilization at wrist, forearm, elbow, shoulder, spine, scapula, and hand
- Manual therapy of muscle energy, myofascial release, and indirect inherent force types
- Specific strengthening of abdominal and scapular stabilizers
- Iontophoresis
- Occasional use of foam roller to assist with spinal extension in the thoracic region

Sessions combined these and lasted approximately 1 hour each for a total of 14 visits over 8 weeks. An integrated upper extremity movement awareness exercise done side lying was used during the whole time to allow her an opportunity to assess her movement capabilities, limitations, and become more confident in her ability to do the home exercise program that developed as they learned what worked best for her. Much effort was required to help the patient see the need to slow down and notice small differences in how she moved, become aware of the way the different movements felt, and develop a sense of internal rightness about posture and control of movement.

It was not until nearly the end of the treatment process that the patient was able to learn how to be subjectively aware enough to perform self-assessment and be independent with specific exercises for balancing and restoring the correct relationships between the muscles and joints from core central axis to the hand. All members of the team agreed in retrospect that this ability to be aware and sense the internal rightness of posture and position was the single most important aspect of this patient's successful outcome. Her improvements came in phases, and seemed to be especially related to when she was able to discontinue a holding of tension pattern within the postural muscles involved. This occurred first in the central musculature and moved to the periphery gradually. As the postural muscles relaxed, the pain decreased, and she became stronger without need for specific repetitive strengthening with weights or bands. The release of held tension in postural muscles appeared to allow a balancing of forces that created more efficiency in the dynamic muscles of the upper quarter.

As her ability to assess her own movement patterns and release the tension in the involved areas by means of self-mobilizations and stretches using enhancers such as gravity and breathing improved, she was able to gradually increase her practice and performance times to previous levels of intensity by the end of the second month. She has remained pain-free and fully functional since that time, now 3 years in length. The course of improvement continued for many months following the end of therapy. Her observation was that the improvements in posture and shoulder position and stability were the most important part of her recovery. An added benefit was more confidence in her own sense of internal control, which then manifested as better posture. She relates that people started asking her if she had lost weight, which prompted her to then actually try and succeed in losing weight. Her internal state underwent a transformation that resulted in a clearly discernable change in her outward appearance.

Looking retrospectively at this case, the element that seems most important is the importance of the relationships. These include those between the musician, therapist, physician, and teacher and the ones within the patient's own body. The communication to the musician that she has a body that can heal, that there are many ways to get to the desired result, and that therapy needs to be individualized for her needs is absolutely essential. Her participation and involvement are essential. The ability of the supporting cast to listen to the patient and each other and then adapt their therapeutic tools to fit her needs is important. There is not a simple answer to these problems, because they involve the way the musician has or has not adapted to her environment. Adaptation involves changes in both sensory integration and motor planning. The take-home point for the caregiver is to listen first, find out what has gotten in the way of the ability to support normal function, help the musician remove the obstacles to healing, and find his or her way back to the uniquely skilled ability he or she has to perform. Specific comments by the therapist about what seemed most important in this case were the time and patience required to help teach internal proprioceptive awareness. Progressing as with children in neurodevelopmental sequencing, patients are taught to listen for the subtle internal changes and little movement pattern changes until they finally get it. Their ability to sense this is the most important thing! Many patients don't get in touch with anything inside at first. To do this requires the use of smaller movement patterns, breathing techniques, letting go of older patterns, so that they can get a sense of something different going on. As an example, pelvic floor stabilization is often required in order for the patient to be able to have a foundation for scapular stabilization, which is necessary for the normal muscular patterns needed for bowing with the upper extremity. People are so sympathetically driven, it is hard to slow them down enough to pay attention to small differences in movement, or learn how to use the breath to quiet physiologically. As in pediatric rehabilitation, midrange movement patterns are emphasized, and the therapist keeps the patient in mid-range and cues with the hands. It is helpful to use visual metaphors to give them ideas about how to move and employ interactive patience, as when learning to dance.

Components of a therapeutic relationship with musicians

To summarize, the authors suggest these components are of primary importance in caring for this special population.

Validation

People need the caregiver to be able to see what it is they are experiencing and understand to some degree how it feels. That is the point of engagement, where the relationship is able to begin.

Space

This is a place where people can discuss without fear of exposure or retribution the physical and emotional aspects of their problem and be heard by someone who has the ability to assist them.

Time

Individuals need time to formulate a description of their experience of the problem, develop a sense of its meaning within the context of their life, and be allowed to hear their own version of the story. This requires silence on the part of the listener. Listening is a practice that is difficult and sometimes even dangerous. Deep attentive listening has the power to draw one into the mystery called silence. Often in listening, one encounters other people and one's own life in new ways [24].

Understanding the problem

What is it? How does it cause a problem with the way the body works? This is more difficult than it sounds. First of all, what are the differences in the way it is perceived by the artist and how it is perceived by the physician? Are there barriers to them speaking the same language? The doctor has a better chance teaching the patient about the body and its route back to normal function if the doctor understands the way it feels for the musician to be in his or her body. That can be a beginning. It shifts the treatment of a condition from something out there administered by doctors to a perspective on how to work from within himself or herself to best cope with a disease or disorder that has taken away his or her vitality. In the journey that follows, the artist needs to be able to see himself or herself as a whole person capable of the return to normal function to negotiate the many steps that may be involved.

The ability for the caregiver to provide and the artist to receive
the needed treatment

Therapies are not just something given by one person and passively received by another. They are an interactive dance, much like the performance of an ensemble. Engagement and the presence of both persons are required. There is give and take of information and skills and a transfer of knowledge, both in the way of the mind and in the way of the body. What does it feel like to move one's arm this way, and how is it different than that way?

The ability of the caregiver to initiate and negotiate referrals to other
doctors, therapists, and treatment/test procedures if/as needed

This is a sensitive task that requires finesse. It is an art. Skill is developed over time as one practices within a community. For each individual patient, trying to choreograph the interplay of personalities, sequence of events, balancing the patient's need to participate and to receive, is a dance. It involves talking about what to expect, what might happen at the visit, how to prepare for it, and what possible options are available for treatment. If one knows the patient well, the doctor can introduce him or her to the network of people available in the community who can help best. The health care system is scary for patients. It is a foreign land, and it does not feel safe.

The ability of music teachers to listen to, and respect the needs
of, the music student in a holistic way, collaborating with others involved
in the student's care

This requires that the teacher take the long view of a student's musical journey. He or she must help the student select short-term achievable goals for musical growth while facilitating recovery.

The ability of the artist to assimilate and incorporate the effect
and meaning of the treatment(s) into himself or herself and continue
to be an artist

Healing from an illness can be tricky. Can the artist go from injury to impairment to understanding to engagement to transformation into something other than what was before, and yet reformulate himself or herself in a way that allows him or her to continue to be an artist? Is that the way of art? It takes hold of people, and they struggle to understand it, learn it, and become a part of it. Like the clay on the potters' wheel, people are formed into something new. In doing this, they become part of the body of work in their field, which in turn gives them the opportunity to offer something back, perhaps to create something new within their field. Sometimes seemingly unfortunate things like injuries change people, and they find the need to do things differently, because they understand themselves differently. The context of understanding may have widened as a result of the illness, and so one sees another way to be about or do work that was previously not within his or her repertoire. This creative act can be a gift back to the community that changes its course for the better. This is the process by which paradigm shifts change the culture of a field of endeavor.

References

[1] Horvath K. Muscleship: the overlooked foundational element of stringed instrument performance technique. American String Teacher 2003;53(3):68–73.

[2] Harrison C, Paull B. The athletic musician. Lanham (MD): Scarecrow Press; 1997.

[3] Harman S. The evolution of performing arts medicine. In: Sataloff RT, Brandfonbrener AG, Lederman RJ, editors. Performing arts medicine. 2nd edition. San Diego (CA): Singular; 1998. p. 1–18.

[4] Steinhausen F. Die Physiology der Bogenführung. Leipzig (Germany): Breitkopf and Härtel; 1903.

[5] Auer L. Violin playing as I teach it. Philadelphia: J.B. Lippincott; 1960.

[6] Rainbow E. Instrumental music: recent research and considerations for future investigations. Bulletin for the Council for Research in Music Education 1973;33:8–31.

[7] Rolland P, Mutschler M. The teaching of action in string playing. Urbana (IL): Illinois String Research Associates; 1986.

[8] Fishbein M, Middlestadt SE, Ottati V, et al. Medical problems among ICSOM musicians: overview of a national survey. Med Probl Perform Art 1988;3(1):1–8.

[9] Horvath J. Playing (less) hurt, revised edition. Kearney (NE): Morris Publishing; 2004.

[10] Wilson FR, Roehmann FL. The study of biomechanical and physiological processes in relation to musical performance. In: Colwell R, editor. The handbook of research on music teaching and learning. New York: Schirmer Books; 1992. p. 509–24.

[11] Brandfonbrener AG, Lederman RJ. Performing arts medicine. In: Colwell R, Richardson C, editors. The new handbook of research on music teaching and learning. New York: Oxford University Press; 2002. p. 1009–22.

[12] Chesky K, Kondraske GV, Henoch M, et al. Musicians' health. In: Colwell R, Richardson C, editors. The new handbook of research on music teaching and learning. New York: Oxford University Press; 2002. p. 1023–39.

[13] National Association of Schools of Music. Handbook 2005–6. Available at: http://nasm. arts-accredit.org. Accessed March 25, 2006.

[14] Health Promotion in Schools of Music. Purpose of the conference. Available at: www.unt. edu/hpsm. Accessed March 19, 2006.

[15] Chesky K. Health Promotion in Schools of Music. HPSM conference program book. Denton (TX): University of North Texas; 2004.

[16] Health Promotion in Schools of Music. NASM: professional health recommendations for framework and practice. Available at: www.unt.edu/hpsm. Accessed April 13, 2006.

[17] Fox M, Sheldrake R. Natural grace: dialogues on creation, darkness, and the soul in spiri-
      tuality and science. New York: Image Books Doubleday; 1996.
[18] Muller W. How, then, shall we live? Four simple questions that reveal the beauty and mean-
      ing of our lives. New York: Bantam Books; 1996.
[19] Muller W. Legacy of the heart: the spiritual advantages of a painful childhood. New York:
      Simon and Shuster; 1992.
[20] Muller W. Sabbath: finding rest, renewal, and delight in our busy lives. New York: Bantam
      Books; 1999.
[21] Heller S. Too loud, too bright, too fast, too tight: what to do if you are sensory defensive in an
      overstimulating world. New York: Harper Collins; 2002.
[22] Kranowitz CS. The out-of-sync child: recognizing and coping with sensory processing disor-
      der, revised and updated edition. New York: The Berkley Publishing Group; 2005.
[23] Butler DS. The sensitive nervous system. Adelaide (Australia): Noigroup Publications; 2000.
[24] Saliers D, Saliers E. A song to sing, a life to live: reflections on music as spiritual practice.
      San Francisco (CA): Jossey-Bass; 2005.

ELSEVIER
SAUNDERS

Phys Med Rehabil Clin N Am
17 (2006) 893–903

PHYSICAL MEDICINE
AND REHABILITATION
CLINICS OF
NORTH AMERICA

Assessing the Instrumentalist Interface: Modifications, Ergonomics and Maintenance of Play

Seneca A. Storm, MD

Michigan State University College of Osteopathic Medicine, Department of Physical Medicine and Rehabilitation, B401 West Fee Hall, East Lansing, MI 48824, USA

"Part of the beauty of making music is that it can be done for decades. There are numerous examples of outstanding instrumentalists who have performed well into their 80s and 90s. Individuals should be encouraged to continue to perform and even to learn to play an instrument late in life. The joy of performing, either for oneself or for others, is not precluded by age" [1].

Approaching the musculoskeletal system of the instrumentalist as it relates to play of their instrument presents a variety of unique challenges. Certainly, similarities exist between the risk of injury resulting from repetitive behaviors performed in industry or while playing an instrument. Musicians behave differently than injured workers in the worker's compensation system, however. Performing artists also draw comparisons to athletes. Consider that some may have hypermobility, some may have short fifth fingers or lack independent sublimis control of the fourth and fifth digits. Effective evaluation starts with knowledge and understanding how the instrument is played, observing techniques, and determining if a change in fit, function, or guidelines for playtime may preserve the ability to play into late life.

Many factors may be involved in the development of injury in the instrumentalist. The physician and health care providers caring for the instrumentalist must identify activities that may be worsening a complaint to determine whether there may be modifications that may facilitate decrease in symptoms. Although instruments are not the same, there are similarities in principle and concepts common chores of supporting the instruments, repetitive key depression, instrument maintenance, and tuning. In addition, individual anatomic variation may influence the interface of the instrumentalist with their chosen instrument. When obtaining history from the instrumentalist, one

E-mail address: seneca.storm@ht.msu.edu

1047-9651/06/$ - see front matter © 2006 Elsevier Inc. All rights reserved.
doi:10.1016/j.pmr.2006.08.003

must consider other instruments, hobbies, and physical activities that may be the source of or contributing to a particularly pain complaint [2].

Reports of musculoskeletal injuries in instrumentalists range from 32% to 78% [3]. Although it has been observed that musicians who start playing at younger ages are older when they present with playing-related complaints, musician's lives involve fluctuations for a variety of reasons. The development of injuries has been associated with an abrupt increase in practice time [4,5]. Classical and nonclassical instruments are associated with a variety of painful conditions in the upper extremities. Overuse syndrome, tendonitis, nerve entrapments, focal dystonia, exertional compartment syndromes, and osteoarthritis are among the differential for pain complaints in the forearm and hand of the instrumentalist. The application of many cycles of stress in the "physiologic" joint range eventually leads to overuse injury when the microtrauma exceeds the adaptive ability [6]. Sometimes a precise diagnosis can be established, but understanding the physical demands of playing an instrument along with ergonomic considerations may provide simple solutions.

Managing symptoms demands consideration of patterns observed in different instruments. The human body is incredibly adaptable, and as we learn from work related to deconditioning, joints, ligaments and muscles are developed and maintained according to activities commonly practiced. Many professional musicians start playing at an early age. As they grow, their anatomy may reflect their instruments [7]. Similarly, as they age, they may accommodate their playing to degenerative joint changes that allow them to continue to play in their advancing years [8]. Understanding the complaints of a musician requires not only evaluation of the patient, but also observation of the musician playing their instrument as well as discussion with music teachers. Discussion of technique and related posture may be delicate discussions, but they are important to understanding how the individual plays. Although one can presume that "perfect" technique might eliminate the risk of injury, this is not the case. Importantly, an "imperfect" or individual technique may not interfere with success or maintenance of play. Vladimir Horowitz played piano with virtually flat, extended fingers and, of note, played with remarkable facility until he died, not showing external stigma of degenerative joint disease in his hands [9].

Establishing tasks required for play of the instrument, developing an understanding of techniques, obtaining practice history and schedules, and determining instruments played, hobbies, and activities not related to play all assist in the assessment of the instrumentalist. Recent and resolved past musculoskeletal complaints may have led to altered technique and secondary injury. Regardless of whether we are personally familiar with all the variations in technique and details of playing a particular instrument, we can develop an approach to understanding the demands through general principles and communication with the instrumentalists and their teachers.

Instruments frequently encountered in orchestras and marching bands may be more familiar to most physicians. A good internet resource for traditional musical instruments is *http://larkinthemorning.com*, which boasts that it is the world's largest selection of ethnic musical instruments. Some traditional instruments appear like evolutionary precursors of guitars, others have no equivalent. This does not mean that the instrumentalists are injury free. A study of Iranian instrumentalists playing the Daf or the setar found greater rates of cumulative trauma disorders than the investigators expected [10]. Although the setar is similar to a guitar, there is no equivalent to the Daf.

In evaluating a particular instrument, we must consider the posture that the player maintains while playing, how the weight of the instrument is supported, repetitive tasks involved in playing the instrument, and pressure points between the instrument and the player. Lastly, when considering wind instruments, we must consider the contact and physiologic effort involved in sound production. Our discussion of a few individual instruments will help illustrate these concepts.

Posture and musculoskeletal complaints

Many instruments require awkward postures involved in playing a particular instrument, often at the end range of motion of a joint. This may increase loading on the musculoskeletal system and increased joint moments or postural asymmetry, all of which may lead to symptoms [11]. Back strain may result from asymmetric playing postures. The tendency toward counterclockwise rotation of the spine in the guitarist facilitates right shoulder protraction and placement of the strumming hand. Widening the strap can help decrease the tension on the left trapezius and periscapular muscles.

Evaluation of the whole body must be taken into account, starting with whether the instrument is played in a seated position, which may limit the ability to move around freely. An instrument typically played in the seated position is the piano. Keyboardists have a high incidence of overuse injuries and reports of pain in their upper back, neck and shoulders. Schools of piano technique abound, with different recommendations about wrist and finger position. Generally, keyboards are played in the seated position, elbows flexed, with wrists near neutral with varying degrees of finger flexion.

Playing the flute requires a tilted and rotated head position. Prolonged static muscle contractions may lead to early degenerative changes in the cervical spine and contribute to right shoulder girdle muscles. The tilted and rotated position may worsen symptoms of cervical radiculitis by mechanical compression over time. Adaptations to the flute include the mouthpiece made by Emerson Musical Instruments in Elkhart, Indiana. The mouthpiece has a 30° obtuse angle just past the lip plate, thereby allowing a near-neutral posture [11]. Violinists commonly develop myofascial pain symptoms in the trapezius and cervical spine muscles. They may also develop worsening symptoms from the cervical spine with foraminal impingement leading to radiculitis.

Shoulders and elbows have relatively confined range of motion when playing many woodwind, brass, and stringed instruments. Wrist position varies in degree of flexion with additional radial or ulnar deviation, while fingers operate strings and keys. Sometimes this is an asymmetric task. In the case of the right-handed guitar, there is increased radial deviation on the left hand and ulnar deviation of the picking/strumming hand. Bass guitarists also have a position of increased radial deviation in the left hand and increased wrist flexion on the right hand. Analysis of posture in the guitarist should also include evaluation of the impact zone of the edge of the guitar top with the elbow region on the picking hand.

String instruments may be bowed, strummed, or picked. Typically, the right hand is involved in handling the bow or holding a plectrum. Consideration of the bow hand and the variations in technique are beyond the scope of our discussion but may be relevant to pain complaints. Maintaining the plectrum between the thumb and second digit in the right hand during guitar playing may lead to stress at the thumb joint. Alternately, the guitar may be strummed with the bare hand, or finger picks may be used.

Size of instrument

The size of the instrument and its fit with the individual instrumentalist may play a role in injury. In studying violists, Blum found that playing a larger instrument led to increased rates of injury, regardless of the musician's size [12]. The International Conference of Symphony and Opera Musicians (ICSOM) survey in 1985 found that with increasing size of string instrument, rates of injury increased in women. Generally, the occurrence of injury is greater in women than men [13].

Instruments and their players come in all shapes and sizes. Hauling instruments to and from practices and performances may significantly aggravate or exacerbate injury or lead to pain-induced modifications, which may predispose to possible nonplaying-related injury. Proper lifting mechanics are always advisable. Using hand trucks and cases on wheels can help and should be encouraged if not done already.

Playing an instrument that is "too large" for the player often leads to extreme postures and resultant injury. This example is truest in young children. In some cases, a smaller instrument may be available. This is particularly true of violins, which come in a variety of sizes. Another example of a modification can allow the child to access all of the buttons by bringing the body of the flute closer. There is great variability in the size and shape of guitars, and, although scientific study has not found an association in style of guitar and development of musculoskeletal injury, the size and shape of the guitar played and the chosen height of the guitar on the guitarist deserves careful consideration. Kopfstein-Penk [14] suggests that the size of the guitar be matched to the guitarist's anthropometric measurements [11].

Consideration of the right forearm pronation and wrist flexion and the left forearm supination and wrist flexion can help determine effect of size of guitar body and position of guitar on the player. While strumming a right-handed guitar, the right shoulder is protracted and internally rotated, and pressure at the elbow may lead to ulnar nerve irritation. The lower "bout" of the acoustic guitar (the part of the guitar body where the right forearm crosses the instrument) may have a beveled edge to alleviate this pressure.

Instrument maintenance

Generally, care of the instrument may reduce the effort required to play. Professional pianists become skilled at controlling the depression of keys in such a way that a professional pianist can play aggressively and decelerate such that the finger does not bang against the end-point. This is a form of learned joint protection. A correlation with injury has been shown with increased pressure and strain on the keys of the keyboard. Changing instruments, particularly if the force a musician has become accustomed to applying to depress the keys suddenly leads to pounding the interphalangeal (IP) joint, may precipitate injury even if both instruments are keyboard related. Traveling pianists may be at particular risk for injury because they play on different instruments, which may be more or less responsive.

Careful maintenance of instruments may limit the effort required to depress keys or strings. String instruments can be altered for ease of play. Alteration of the bridge can change the distance the fingers of the left hand must depress the string. Changing to a lower string gauge may also help reduce the tension experienced while playing, although a change in tone may occur. Tuning instruments and changing the strings can lead to awkward positions, which may exacerbate injury. This is particularly true of the harp.

Key modifications allow easy accommodation for a variety of instruments including the flute, clarinet, oboe, saxophone, and bassoon to allow a better fit to the patient's hand. Some portion of the population has a short fifth digit. As a result, reaching some standard keys is difficult. Examples would be the extended A key on the flute, or lengthening the C# key on the oboe for a short fifth finger may allow the patient to reach the key without bending the wrist [15].

Support of the instrument

Depending on the type of instrument, the musician may be required to support part or all of the weight of the instrument. Playing an instrument requires static and dynamic loads on the musculoskeletal system. A static load required for playing an instrument is continuous muscle contraction with stress across a joint and its supporting structures. How the instrument is supported, whether the weight is born through a strap, positions of the neck, shoulders, elbows, and wrists should be evaluated. Musculoskeletal loading as it relates to the instrument against a body part or the overall weight of the instrument also needs consideration.

Static loading, sometimes in awkward postures, as well as the dynamic components of playing each individual instrument should be considered. Stress to the joints and their supporting structures during movement, typically a high-frequency, repetitive movement, is a dynamic load. The dynamic load of an instrument may be altered by regular maintenance, string gauge, and bridge location (which influences the distance strings must be moved during play).

For the violinist, the left shoulder is placed under static load, and the right shoulder experiences both dynamic and static loading. String and wind instrumentalists are particularly inclined toward shoulder problems as the joint is often under these prolonged static and dynamic loads.

When considering prolonged periods spent playing an instrument, we can learn from effects of immobilization on joints. Prolonged positioning of the elbow at 90° can lead to shortening of the elbow flexors and lengthening of the elbow extensors. Although playing may not have the same risks as immobilization, prolonged static positions may lead to relative immobilization of joints.

Woodwind and brass instruments involve the production of air from the body in contact with the instrument. In evaluation of any instrument, we must consider how the body supports the instrument. We must evaluate how the right and left hands are involved in the movements. Although both hands might be in operation of the instrument, there may be static support and dynamic activity involving the same hand.

In the case of the saxophone, the instrument is held out in the frontal plane of the body. The addition of the neck strap has been helpful for the alto and tenor saxophones. Chest straps may be useful for the baritone saxophone player. Chest straps may help decrease the choking effect that may be felt with the neck strap. Despite the use of straps, some portion of the instrument weight may be born through the hands. Forces at the tip of the thumb may be transmitting compressive forces to the base. This may exacerbate degenerative joint disease at the thumb joint, and it may be wise to minimize activities where the thumb acts as a lever [2]. Degenerative problems in the thumb can be most troubling in performing artists. The trapeziometacarpal "saddle" articulation allows for significant mobility, which also predisposes this joint to disabling degeneration. The thumb position required for performing a "thumb under" maneuver at the piano or while holding the large bow of the double bass or cello leads to great compressive forces. The basal joint is subjected to 12 times the forces, and the metacarpophalangeal joint six times the forces for each kilogram of force transmitted through the tip of the thumb [16].

Many instruments require that the musician support the weight of the instrument while applying rapid sequences of finger motion in the upper extremities. In many instruments, the right thumb bears the weight of much of this support. There is a chronic stretch applied to the right thumb meta-carpophalangeal joints, particularly in heavier instruments. Over time, with prolonged, intense practice, the weight of a two-pound clarinet may contribute to chronic pain. A shelf deformity may develop in patients complaining of pain who have a long-standing history of supporting the weight of their instrument on their thumbs. The flute supports the weight primarily through the left thumb. As musicians age, particularly, the years of this chore may lead to digital neuritis, or arthritis of the CMC joint might progress, and broadening the support may decrease symptoms in the left thumb. Making changes to pad support as well as key movement and modification to allow for more natural hand position may improve symptoms.

In an attempt to decrease the weight of the instrument on the patient, many instruments have been adapted. Modified microphone stands may support the oboe, chair stands can stabilize and support the clarinet, and there are stands to support the weight of a bass. Some musicians may choose to use the support only when they are practicing. Individual modification of instruments is limited only by a player's creativity.

The viola de gamba, the predecessor to the cello, is held between the knees of the musician. The addition of the Stahlhammer or angled end-pin allowed the musician to balance the instrument instead of wholly support it. End pins can be used with the English horn, the bass, the oboe, and the tuba. For the bassoon, a seat strap may help support the weight of the instrument.

The accordion may weigh up to 40 pounds and may lead to back problems despite the use of straps. A back strap should always be used and lifting the instrument into position may contribute to back discomfort. More information is available about Accordions at *www.ksanti.net/free-reed/*. An example of modifications made by a concertina player to relieve his symptoms is available online at *www.concertina.net/kc_ortho.html/*.

Attempts to alter the support of any instrument must also take into account patient technique, which may be difficult or impossible to modify. In the case of the violin, the support should act to decrease the amount of pressure required to secure the instrument between the mandible and the trapezius. An example of this sort of design is the Voelskow shoulder rest. In addition, the size and weight of the stringed instrument may contribute to shoulder pain. Blum and colleagues [12] found that violists who played larger instruments (>40 cm) had a greater tendency toward shoulder pain.

Consideration of hypermobility in the instrumentalist

Hypermobility refers to joint laxity. Several criteria exist to establish a diagnosis of hypermobility. One such set of criteria is the Beighton scoring system:

1. Place hands flat on the floor with knees extended (1 point).

2. Apposition of the thumb to the flexor surface of the forearm (1 point per side).
3. Hyperextension of the fifth digit to 90° (1 point per side).
4. Hyperextension of the knee beyond 190° (1 point per side).
5. Hyperextension of the elbow beyond 190° (1 point per side).

Using the Beighton scoring system, generalized hypermobility is determined if a score of four or more of nine points is assigned [17]. Whether hypermobility affords a relative advantage or disadvantage to the instrumentalist is the subject of great debate. Brandfonbrener [18] has noted that women have higher rates of hypermobility and higher rates of injuries than male counterpoints in their survey.

Larsson and coworkers [19] explored what advantages might be found in subjects with hypermobility/hyperlaxity of their joints. Although they found joint hypermobility was beneficial in joint subjected to repetitive motion of playing, but detrimental to joints subject to static loads. Because most instruments require static loading, patients with hypermobility may be at increased risk for injury.

Careful evaluation of individual joints in the hand may allow for construction of a supporting orthotics, which may provide some increased stability in the case of a symptomatic hypermobile joint. In evaluating joint hypermobility, it may be helpful to have the patients "warm up" because joint range of motion may increase substantially after training and "warm up." Adaptive devices may be used to limit the likelihood of spontaneous dislocation [20].

Musicians with disabilities

Disability does not interfere with the individual desire for creative expression, nor does it interfere with the experience and potential benefits. Music and performing arts history offer examples of artists afforded unique perspective perhaps, in part, by way of their impairments. One report of blind musicians found that they had a greater prevalence of absolute pitch than do their sighted peers [21].

Another great resource is http://www.vsarts.org. VSA arts, formerly known as very special arts, is an affiliate of the John F. Kennedy Center for Performing Arts. Their mission is to "create and enjoy the arts". This site has links to a variety of sites aimed at adaptive equipment as well as art supplies and adaptive tools for everything from head painting to motorized easels. Other interesting links include Arts as a source of healing, building, and empowerment (http://artlynx.org) and A Day's Work: Designing and constructing musical instruments and adaptive aids for professionals and their students or clients in: Music Education, Music Therapy, Special Education, Occupational Therapy and Elder Care. Another site for general adaptive equipment, http://www.sammonspreston.com may be useful in joint protection and is a good resource for practitioners to review as well.

While each patient handles the trauma, loss, and recovery of a disabling event in their own time, may examples exist of musicians who have incorporated their changed or changing bodies into their style of play. In an increasingly digital age, voice-to-midi/midi keyboards allow for musical expression, and a variety of resources are available. In the pursuit of artistic expression, the only insurmountable obstacle is lack of imagination. Curtis Mayfield is a well-known example of a guitar player/musician who determined that he would continue making music after a stage accident resulted in quadriplegia. The stories available through www.paralinks.com tell accounts of individual artists who have found ways to continue making music. Another site with good information is the Coalition for musicians with disabilities, http://www.disabled-musicians.org. Technologies are available for controlling 128 instruments, various beats, vocals, and chords while using whatever movement a patient can best control. Information is available at http://www.switchintime.com.

Summary

Awareness of the tasks required to play a particular instrument requires observation of technique and understanding of the dynamic and static loads placed on the musculoskeletal system to play a particular instrument. Anatomic differences, variation in hand size, gender, instrument choice, and maintenance of the instrument all may play a role in the development of playing-related complaints. Simply observing particular instruments, we can see a variety of positions that are required to play the instrument. Important to the discussion of overuse syndromes, we must evaluate the duration of practice sessions and warm-up and cool down periods, which may help minimize playing-related problems. Avoid absolute rest and opt for relative rest for playing-related problems. Immobilization for more than 3 to 4 weeks may lead to greater risk of injury when playing is resumed. Return to play schedules should start with simple, soft music, doubling minutes of playing every few days, dropping back if pain develops [22] Practical advice may include building up practice times gradually with 5- to 10-minute intervals in 60- to 90-minutes sessions [23]. This recommendation is supported by the findings of Lutz and colleagues [24] who showed decreased blood flow to the forearm after repetitive hand and wrist activities for 90 minutes. This decrease in blood flow normalized after 5 to 10 minutes of stretching exercises. Players with hypermobility should consider limiting practice sessions to 45 minutes allowing for rest breaks of 10 to 15 minutes [20].

Fry [25] suggested a shift in thinking of ergonomics as a reactive strategy to one in which we anticipate and prevent problems before they become insidious or severe enough to limit the ability of the instrumentalist to play. Joint protection is important in all musicians, and although youth can be forgiving for many, we must remind our patients about joint protection as it applies to activities of daily living. Instrumentalists rely on their hands and finger joints to allow them to perform. Basic principles that apply to patients with all types of arthritis also apply to our patients when activities that worsen symptoms or place unnecessary stress on joints are identified. Using adaptive equipment to open jars is an obvious example. Overall, engaging the patient to observe routine behaviors may lead to the identification of modifiable activities, which might be aggravating or manifesting as a playing-related discomfort. Although some injury patterns can be associated with particular instruments, remember that your guitar-playing patient may be taking drum lessons on the side, which could result in lateral epicondylitis that bothers him when he plays the guitar.

References

[1] Hoppmann RA, Ekman EF. Arthritis in the aging musician. Med Probl Perform Art 1999; 14(2):80.
[2] Hoppmann R. Musculoskeletal problems in instrumental musicians. In: Sataloff RT, Brandfonbrener AG, Lederman RJ, editors. Performing arts medicine. 2nd edition. San Diego (CA): Singular; 1998. p. 205–30.
[3] Fishbein M, Middlestadt SE, Ottai V, et al. Medical problems among ICSOM musicians: overview of a national survey. Med Probl Perform Art 1988;3:1–8.
[4] Fry H. Prevalence of overuse (injury) syndrome in Australian music schools. Br J Ind Med 1987;44:35–40.
[5] Newmark J, Lederman R. Practice doesn't necessarily make perfect: incidence of overuse syndromes in amateur instrumentalists. Med Probl Perform Art 1987;2:142–4.
[6] Pitner M. Pathophysiology of overuse injuries in the hand and wrist. Hand Clin 1990;6(3): 355–63.
[7] Beijani FJ, Kaye GM, Henham M. Musculoskeletal and neuromuscular conditions of instrumental musicians. Arch Phys Med Rehabil 1996;77:406–13.
[8] Barton R. The aging musician. Work 2004;22(2):131–8.
[9] Brandfonbrener A. The etiologies of medical problems in performing artists in performing arts medicine. 2nd edition. San Diego (CA): Singular; 1998. p. 19–40.
[10] Sadeghi S, Kazemi B, Shooshtari S, et al. A high prevalence of cumulative trauma disorders in Iranian instrumentalists. BMC Musculoskelet Disord 2004;5:35.
[11] Norris R, Dommerholt J. Applied ergonomics: adaptive equipment and instrument modification for musicians. In: Sataloff RT, Brandfonbrener AG, Lederman RJ, editors. Performing Arts Medicine. 2nd edition. San Diego (CA): Singular; 1998. p. 261–75.
[12] Blum JAJ. Ergonomic considerations in violists' left shoulder pain. Med Probl Perform Art 1994;9:25–9.
[13] Middlestadt S, Fishbein M. The prevalence of severe musculoskeletal problems among male and female symphony orchestra string players. Med Probl Perform Art 1989;4: 41–8.
[14] Kopfstein-Penk A. The Healthy Guitar: finding a guitar that reduces injury risk and improves your playing. Arlington, VA: MMB Music; 1994.
[15] Blatt R. Preventing overuse injuries in oboists. The Double Reed Spring 1990;13(2):64–5.
[16] Barron O, Eaton RG. The upper limb of the performing artist. In: Sataloff RT, Brandfonbrener AG, Lederman RJ, editors. Performing arts medicine. 2nd edition. San Diego (CA): Singular; 1998. p. 231–60.
[17] Beighton P, Solomon L, Soskoine C. Articular mobility in an African population. Ann Rheum Dis 1973;32:413–8.
[18] Brandfonbrener A. Joint laxity in instrumental musicians. Med Probl Perform Art 1990;5: 117–9.

[19] Larrson L, Baum J, Mudholkar GS. Hypermobility: features and differential incidence between the sexes. Arthritis Rheum 1987;30:1426–30.
[20] Hoppmann RAPN. Musculoskeletal problems in instrumental musicians. In: Textbook of Performing Arts Medicine. New York: Singular; 1991. p. 71–100.
[21] Hamilton RHP-LA, Schlaug G. Absolute pitch in blind musicians. Neuroreport 2004;15(5): 803–6.
[22] Warrington J. Hand therapy for the musician: instrument-focused rehabilitation. Hand Clin 2003;19:287–301.
[23] Amadio P, Russotti G. Evaluation and treatment of hand and wrist disorders in musicians. Hand Clinics 1990;6(3):405–16.
[24] Lutz G, Hansford T. CTD controls: the ergonomics program at Ethicon, Inc. J Hand Surg 1987;12A:863.
[25] Fry H. The treatment of overuse injury syndrome. Maryland Med J 1993;42(3):277–82.

ELSEVIER
SAUNDERS

Phys Med Rehabil Clin N Am
17 (2006) 905–910

PHYSICAL MEDICINE
AND REHABILITATION
CLINICS OF
NORTH AMERICA

Index

Note: Page numbers of article titles are in **boldface** type.

1047-9651/06/$ - see front matter © 2006 Elsevier Inc. All rights reserved.
doi:10.1016/S1047-9651(06)00079-9